# Avoiding Errors in
# Adult Medicine

D0551948

## Ian P. Reckle

BSc, MRCP, MBA
Consultant Physician and Assist~ . Medical Director
Oxford University Hospitals NHS Trust
Oxford, UK

## D. John M. Reynolds

DPhil, FRCP
Consultant Physician and Clinical Pharmacologist
Oxford University Hospitals NHS Trust
Oxford, UK

## Sally Newman

BSc, LLM
Solicitor, Head of Legal Services
Oxford University Hospitals NHS Trust
Oxford, UK

## Joseph E. Raine

MD, FRCPCH, DCH
Consultant Paediatrician
Whittington Hospital
London, UK

## Kate Williams

MA (Oxon)
Partner
Radcliffes LeBrasseur Solicitors
Leeds, UK

## Jonathan Bonser

BA (Oxon)
Consultant in the Healthcare Department of
Fishburns LLP, Solicitors
London, UK
Former Head of the Claims and Legal Services
Department of the Leeds office of the Medical Protection Society

## WILEY-BLACKWELL

A John Wiley & Sons, Ltd., Publication

This edition first published 2013 © 2013 by John Wiley & Sons, Ltd.

Wiley-Blackwell is an imprint of John Wiley & Sons, formed by the merger of Wiley's global Scientific, Technical and Medical business with Blackwell Publishing.

*Registered office:*  John Wiley & Sons, Ltd, The Atrium, Southern Gate, Chichester, West Sussex, PO19 8SQ, UK

*Editorial offices:*  9600 Garsington Road, Oxford, OX4 2DQ, UK
The Atrium, Southern Gate, Chichester, West Sussex, PO19 8SQ, UK
111 River Street, Hoboken, NJ 07030-5774, USA

For details of our global editorial offices, for customer services and for information about how to apply for permission to reuse the copyright material in this book please see our website at www.wiley.com/wiley-blackwell

*Library of Congress Cataloging-in-Publication Data*

Avoiding errors in adult medicine / Ian P. Reckless ... [et al.].
       p. ; cm.
   Includes bibliographical references and index.
   ISBN 978-0-470-67438-3 (pbk. : alk. paper)
   I. Reckless, Ian.
   [DNLM: 1. Great Britain. National Health Service.    2. Medical Errors–legislation & jurisprudence–Great Britain–Case Reports.    3. Medical Errors–prevention & control–Great Britain–Case Reports.    4. Adult–Great Britain.    5. Liability, Legal–Great Britain–Case Reports.    6. Malpractice–Great Britain–Case Reports.    7. State Medicine–legislation & jurisprudence–Great Britain–Case Reports. WB 100]
   610.28′9–dc23

                                                                        2012031979

A catalogue record for this book is available from the British Library.

Wiley also publishes its books in a variety of electronic formats. Some content that appears in print may not be available in electronic books.

Cover design by Sarah Dickinson Designs

Set in 10.5/13 pt Minion by Aptara® Inc., New Delhi, India
Printed and bound in Malaysia by Vivar Printing Sdn Bhd

1   2013

# Contents

## Part 3  Investigating and dealing with errors

# Contributors

**Joanne Haswell**
Barrister
Director, InPractice Training
London
*Part 3: The role of hospital staff, External investigators, Hospital investigations, The role of the doctor*

**Alistair Hewitt**
Partner, Radcliffes LeBrasseur
Leeds
*Part 3: Coroner's court, Criminal matters*

**Kate Hill**
Solicitor, Radcliffes LeBrasseur
Managing Director, InPractice Training
London
*Part 3: The role of hospital staff, External investigators, Hospital investigations, The role of the doctor*

# Preface

Medical errors in their broadest sense represent a major problem for modern society. It has been estimated that approximately 1 in 10 patients admitted to hospital in the developed world is the victim of an error, and approximately 1 in 300 patients admitted to hospital dies as a result of such an error.

Healthcare professionals tend to act in good faith and medical error has many victims – patients, families, those very medical professionals (and their families) . . .

The spheres of law and medicine overlap increasingly often: human rights; corporate responsibility; NHS standards; rising patient expectations; increasingly complex and ethically challenging interventions; clinical negligence and medical error; and, a compensation culture all collectively create a large amount of work at the medico-legal interface. Physicians and lawyers have each created a language, impenetrable from the outside, with which to conduct their trade – many relatively simple concepts can be lost in translation.

This book aims to help doctors to understand the legal language and concepts, to avoid the major medico-legal traps, and to act promptly and responsibly when errors occur or legal difficulties arise. We hope we have avoided using impenetrable jargon and have been able to present the information in a way that is accessible to all.

The contents of this book inevitably draw on the experience of the authors but by and large, the cases are not directly factual accounts. Where cases do bear relation to real patient stories, any details have been changed sufficiently to fully protect the identities of all involved, other than in the rare case where the information is already firmly within the public domain.

Ian Reckless
D John M Reynolds
Sally Newman

# Abbreviations

| | |
|---|---|
| ACA | Anterior Cerebral Artery |
| AF | Atrial Fibrillation |
| AMU | Acute Medical Unit |
| BNF | British National Formulary |
| BP | Blood Pressure |
| CEMD | Confidential Enquiry into Maternal Death |
| CNS | Central Nervous System |
| CNST | Clinical Negligence Scheme for Trusts |
| CO2 | Carbon Dioxide |
| COPD | Chronic Obstructive Pulmonary Disease |
| CPR | Cardiopulmonary Resuscitation |
| CQC | Care Quality Commission |
| CRP | C-Reactive Protein |
| CSF | Cerebrospinal Fluid |
| CT | Computed Tomography |
| CT1 | Core Trainee (year 1) |
| CT2 | Core Trainee (year 2) |
| CTPA | Computed Tomography Pulmonary Angiogram |
| DNAR | Do Not Attempt Resuscitation |
| DVLA | Driver and Vehicle Licensing Authority |
| ECHR | European Convention on Human Rights |
| ECG | Electrocardiogram |
| ED | Emergency Department |
| EMG | Electromyogram |
| EPA | Enduring Power of Attorney |
| FY1 | Foundation Trainee (year 1) |
| FY2 | Foundation Trainee (year 2) |
| GMC | General Medical Council |
| GP | General Practitioner |
| HSV | Herpes Simplex Virus |
| ICAS | Independent Complaints Advocacy Service |
| IMCA | Independent Mental Capacity Advocate |
| ISQ | In Status Quo |

| | |
|---|---|
| ITU | Intensive Therapy Unit |
| IVF | In Vitro Fertilisation |
| IVIG | Intravenous Immunoglobulin |
| JVP | Jugular Venous Pressure |
| KPa | Kilopascal |
| LBBB | Left Bundle Branch Block |
| LPA | Lasting power of Attorney |
| LFTs | Liver Function Tests |
| M&M | Morbidity and Mortality |
| MCA | Middle Cerebral Artery |
| MCA | Mental Capacity Act 2005 |
| MDT | Multidisciplinary Team |
| MRI | Magnetic Resonance Imaging |
| MRSA | Methicillin Resistant Staphylococcus Aureus |
| NHS | National Health Service |
| NHSLA | National Health Service Litigation Authority |
| NICE | National Institute for Health and Care Excellence |
| OGD | Oesophagogastroduodenoscopy |
| PaO2 | Partial pressure of oxygen in arterial blood |
| PCR | Polymerase Chain Reaction |
| PCT | Primary Care Trust |
| PHSO | Parliamentary and Health Service Ombudsman |
| SHA | Strategic Health Authority |
| SHO | Senior House Officer |
| SIRI | Serious Incident Requiring Investigation |
| SOB | Shortness of Breath |
| SpR | Specialist Registrar |
| ST5 | Specialty Registrar, year 5 |
| TFTs | Thyroid Function Tests |
| TIA | Transient Ischaemic Attack |
| TOE | Transoesophageal echocardiogram |
| UTI | Urinary Tract Infection |
| VP | Ventriculo-peritoneal |
| VTE | Venous Thromboembolism |

# Introduction

In 2000, a committee established by the Department of Health, chaired by the then Chief Medical Officer, Professor Sir Liam Donaldson, published its report *An Organisation with a Memory*. The report recognized that the vast majority of NHS care was of a very high clinical standard and that serious failures were uncommon given the volume of care provided. However, when failures do occur their consequences can be devastating for individual patients and their families. The healthcare workers feel guilt and distress. Like a ripple effect, the errors also undermine the public's confidence in the health service. Last, but not least, these adverse events have a huge cumulative financial effect. Updating the figures provided in the report, in 2010/11, the NHS Litigation Authority (NHSLA, the Special Health Authority body that manages clinical negligence claims against NHS Trusts in England) paid out nearly £863 400 000 for clinical negligence claims (these figures take no account of the costs incurred by claimant and defendant solicitors). The report commented ruefully that often these failures have a familiar ring to them; many could be avoided 'if only the lessons of experience were properly learned'.

The committee writing the report also noted that there is a vast reservoir of clinical data from negligence claims that remains untapped. They were gently critical of the health service as being par excellence a passive learning organization; like a school teacher writing an end-of-term report, they classified the NHS a poor learner – could do better. On a more positive note, the report stated that 'There is significant potential to extract valuable learning by focusing, specialty by specialty, on the main areas of practice that have resulted in litigation.' It acknowledged that learning from adverse clinical events is a key component of clinical governance and is an important component in delivering the government's patient safety and quality agenda for the NHS.

The NHSLA has reported that its present (as of 2011) estimate for all potential liabilities, existing and expected claims, is £16.8 billion. At the time *An Organisation with a Memory* was written, this figure stood at £2.4 billion. (These sums are actuarially calculated figures that are based on both known and as yet unknown claims, some of which may not arise for many years to come. This amount should not be confused with the figure of £863 400 000 mentioned above, which was the sum actually paid out in damages in one calendar year). The NHSLA also reported that the number of clinical negligence claims rose from 6652 in 2009/10 to 8655 in 2010/11 While this may be due to the increased readiness of patients to pursue clinical negligence claims rather than any marked decline in the quality of care provided by the NHS, the statistics clearly show that there is still room for improvement in the care provided to patients. It is this gap in the quality of care that we, the authors, wish to address through this book.

*An Organisation with a Memory* as a report tried to take a fresh look at the nature of adverse events within the NHS. It looked at fields of activity outside healthcare, such as the airline industry. The committee commented that there were two ways of viewing human error: the person-centred approach and the systems approach. The person-centred approach focuses on the individual, his inattention, forgetfulness and carelessness. Its correctives are aimed at individuals and propagate a blame culture. The systems approach, on the other hand, takes a holistic view of the reasons for failure. It recognizes that many of the problems facing large organizations are complex and result from the interplay of many factors: adverse events often arise from the cumulative effect of a number of small errors; they cannot always be pinned on one blameworthy individual. This approach starts from the position that humans do make mistakes and that errors are inevitable, but tries to change the environment in which people work, so that fewer errors will be made.

The systems approach does not, however, absolve individuals of their responsibilities. Rather, it suggests that we should not automatically assume that we should look for an individual to blame for an adverse outcome. The authors of *An Organisation with a Memory* acknowledged that clinical practice did differ from many hi-tech industries. The airline industry, for example, can place a number of hi-tech safeguards between danger and harm. This is often not possible in many fields of clinical practice, where the human elements are often the last and the most important defences. 'In surgery,' they wrote, 'very little lies between the scalpel and some untargeted nerve or blood vessel other than the skill and training of the surgeon.' In addition, healthcare provision is inherently more risky than many hi-tech industries. An airline will suspend flights if conditions are dangerous – physiologically unstable patients cannot always have their treatment suspended simply because they are very sick. Risk-benefit margins are very different in medicine than in aviation. A patient with cancer will inevitably be made to feel ill with aggressive chemotherapy, and they run substantial risks of marrow suppression and other serious adverse effects. The rationale for embarking on high risk treatment is that if untreated the underlying disease is even higher risk. The challenge is to be able to anticipate problems and minimize their impact. We believe that these differences are key to understanding the nature of error in healthcare and they are the reasons why we have placed such great emphasis on case studies that show how doctors make errors in treating their patients.

The committee felt that the NHS had for too long taken a person-centred approach to the errors made by its employees and that this had stifled improvement. They called for a change in the culture of the NHS and a move away from what they saw as its blame culture. More than a decade has passed since the writing of the report and whilst there has been some change in attitudes, more progress is required. We want to see an NHS that promotes a safety culture, rather than a blame culture, a culture where there are multiple safeguards built into the systems of healthcare provision.

However, the legal systems (civil, criminal and coronial) in which the medical services operate do not always foster such an approach. Although coroners can now comment on the strengths and weaknesses of systems in their verdicts, in general, the civil litigation process still tends to focus on the actions of individuals rather than the failings of the healthcare system. Perhaps the most glaring example of this person-centred approach can be seen in the way the General Medical Council treats medical practitioners, when they are notified of concerns about an individual doctor's practice. In that regulatory forum, doctors are expected to meet personal professional standards and will be held to account if they fall short of them in any way. Yet they may find themselves working in an environment that at times seems to conflict with those professional standards.

In Reason (2000), Professor James Reason (originator of the well known 'Swiss Cheese' explanation of how errors sometimes lead to damage) stated:

> The longstanding and widespread tradition of the person approach focuses on the unsafe acts – errors and procedural violations – of people at the sharp end: nurses, physicians, surgeons, anaesthetists, pharmacists, and the like. It views these unsafe acts as arising primarily from aberrant mental processes such as forgetfulness, inattention, poor motivation, carelessness, negligence, and recklessness. Naturally enough, the associated countermeasures are directed mainly at reducing unwanted variability in human behaviour. These methods include poster campaigns that appeal to people's sense of fear, writing another procedure (or adding to existing ones), disciplinary measures, threat of litigation, retraining, naming, blaming, and shaming. Followers of this approach tend to treat errors as moral issues, assuming that bad things happen to bad people – what psychologists have called the just world hypothesis.
>
> The basic premise in the system approach is that humans are fallible and errors are to be expected, even in the best organisations. Errors are seen as consequences rather than causes, having their origins not so much in the perversity of human nature as in 'upstream' systemic factors. These include recurrent error traps in the workplace and the organisational processes that give rise to them. Countermeasures are based on the assumption that though we cannot change the human condition, we can change the conditions under which humans work. A central idea is that of system defences. All hazardous technologies possess barriers and safeguards. When an adverse event occurs, the important issue is not who blundered, but how and why the defences failed. (Reproduced from J. Reason (2000) Human error: models and management, *BMJ* 320:768, with permission from BMJ Publishing Group Ltd.)

As authors, we believe that the committee of *An Organisation with a Memory* were correct, when they wrote that many useful lessons can be learnt from the bitter experience of errors and litigation and that this can best be done by looking specialty by specialty at those areas of medical practice where errors are most frequently made. Thus, we have produced a book looking at errors in adult medicine. It is one of a series of such books, each concentrating on a separate specialty.

If doctors are to learn lessons from their errors and litigation, then they must have some understanding of the underlying processes. Thus, in Part 1, Section 1: Errors and their causes, we discuss types of medical error, the key legal concepts and how they interact with medical practice. In Part 1, Section 2: Medico-legal aspects, we cover the basic legal concepts relevant to medical care: negligence, consent and confidentiality.

The heart of the book is Part 2. Here, we set out a number of case studies on common errors in adult medicine. Each case has its roots in everyday practice and is supplemented with medical and legal comment. Many cases concern failures to diagnose an illness, the commonest source of error in medical treatment.

Finally, Part 3 provides a practical guide to the various forms of concerns that a doctor may encounter, how they may affect him and what he can do to protect his interests.

Our aim is to provide a book that will go some way to meet the challenges laid down at the turn of the millennium in *An Organisation with a Memory*. We hope that it will reduce the number of clinical errors and improve the standard of care provided by individual physicians and hospitals throughout the country.

## References and further reading

Department of Health (2000) An Organisation with a Memory, the report of an expert group on learning from adverse events in the NHS, chaired by the Chief Medical Officer (2000). http://www.dh.gov.uk/en/Publicationsandstatistics/Publications/PublicationsPolicyAndGuidance/DH_4065083.

The National Health Service Litigation Authority Report and Accounts 2010-11. http://www.nhsla.com/NR/rdonlyres/3F5DFA84-2463-468B-890C-42C0FC16D4D6/0/NHSLAAnnualReportandAccounts2011.pdf

Reason J (2000) In human error: models and management. *BMJ* **320**: 768–70.

# PART 1

# Section 1: Errors and their causes

## A few words about error

If our aim is to reduce the number of clinical errors, then we must explain what we mean by 'error'. The Oxford English Dictionary defines 'an error' as a mistake. This is self-evident and does not really help us, the authors, to define our goal.

We could define our aim by looking at the end-result of errors and say that we want to prevent poor patient outcomes. That must be our primary concern, but our aim is broader; many errors can be rectified before any serious harm is done.

We could look at the seriousness of the error, how 'bad' the error actually was. Some errors and their consequences could be so serious that they can be labelled 'criminal' and in fact some cases which fall far short of acceptable standards of practice are investigated by the police and are brought before the criminal courts by the Crown Prosecution Service, as we shall see later. Other errors are the sort that only become obvious with the benefit of hindsight and could be made by anyone, even the best of doctors. In short, we want to look at all errors across the spectrum. What we hope to achieve is to raise the standard of care provided to patients, so that errors of all kinds are reduced.

## Learning from system failures – the vincristine example

The way that the civil courts look at negligence is to focus on the acts of individuals and to ascribe fault to particular actions or omissions of doctors, if their treatment of the patient fell below the standard of the *Bolam* test (see Part 1, Section 2, below). But as mentioned in our Introduction, there is another way of looking at errors and that is to consider system failures.

In order to illustrate the difference between system failures and individual fault, the authors of *An Organisation with a Memory* examined a case concerning the maladministration of the drug vincristine. The case concerns a child but the key learning points are equally applicable to general adult medicine. The mistake cost the patient his life. A number of shortcomings occurred during the patient's stay in the hospital. We believe that it would be useful to set out what happened in the lead up to the patient's death, pointing

*Avoiding Errors in Adult Medicine*, First Edition. Ian P. Reckless, D. John M. Reynolds, Sally Newman, Joseph E. Raine, Kate Williams and Jonathan Bonser.
© 2013 John Wiley & Sons, Ltd. Published 2013 by John Wiley & Sons, Ltd.

out at each stage, the failings that occurred. We will then provide a more detailed discussion of the general lessons that can be learnt from the case.

The following is taken with minor amendment from *An Organisation with a Memory*. It is a classic example of how a number of small errors can add up to a massive error and end with a fatality:

A patient was being treated in a district general hospital (DGH). He was due to receive chemotherapy under a general anaesthetic at a specialist centre. He should have been fasted for 6 hours prior to the anaesthetic, but was allowed to eat and drink before leaving the DGH.

*Fasting error. Poor communication between the DGH and the specialist centre.*

When he arrived at the specialist centre, there were no beds available on the oncology ward, so he was admitted to a mixed-specialty 'outlier' ward.

*Lack of organizational resources; there were no beds available for specialized treatment. The patient was placed in an environment where the staff had no specialist oncology expertise.*

The patient's notes were lost and were not available to the ward staff on admission.

*Loss of patient information.*

The patient was due to receive intravenous vincristine, to be administered by a specialist oncology nurse on the ward, and intrathecal (spinal) methotrexate, to be administered in the operating theatre by an oncology Specialist Registrar. No oncology nurse specialist was available on the ward.

*Communication failure between the oncology department and the outlier ward. Absence of policy and resources to deal with the demands placed on the system by outlier wards, including shortage of specialist staff.*

Vincristine and methotrexate were transported together to the ward by a housekeeper instead of being kept separate at all times.

*Drug delivery error due to noncompliance with hospital policy, which was that the drugs must be kept separate at all times. Communication error: the outlier ward was not aware of this policy.*

The housekeeper who took the drugs to the ward informed staff that both drugs were to go to theatre with the patient.

*Communication error. Incorrect information communicated. Poor delivery practice, allowing drugs to be delivered to outlier wards by inexperienced staff.*

The patient was consented by a junior doctor. He was consented only for intrathecal (IT) methotrexate and not for intravenous vincristine.

*Poor consenting practice. Junior doctor allowed to take consent. Consenting error.*

A junior doctor abbreviated the route of administration to IV and IT, instead of using the full term in capital letters.

*Poor prescribing and documentation practice.*

When the fasting error was discovered, the chemotherapy procedure was postponed from the morning to the afternoon list. The doctor who had been due to administer the intrathecal drug had booked the afternoon off and assumed that another doctor in charge of the wards that day would take over. No formal face-to-face handover was carried out between the two doctors.

*Communication failure. Poor handover of task responsibilities. Inappropriate task delegation.*

The patient arrived in the anaesthetic room and the oncology Senior Registrar was called to administer the chemotherapy. However the doctor was unable to leave his ward and assured the anaesthetist that he should go ahead as this was a straightforward procedure.

*Inadequate protocols regulating the administration of high toxicity drugs. Goal conflict between ward and theatre duties. Poor practice expecting the doctor to be in two places at the same time.*

The oncology Senior Registrar was not aware that both drugs had been delivered to theatre. The anaesthetist had the expertise to administer drugs intrathecally but had never administered chemotherapy. He injected the methotrexate intravenously and the vincristine into the patient's spine. Intrathecal injection of vincristine is almost invariably fatal, and the patient died 5 days later.

*Situational awareness error. Inappropriate task delegation and lack of training. Poor practice to allow chemotherapy drugs to be administered by someone with no oncology experience. Drug administration error.*

Although *An Organisation with a Memory* analyses this sorry tale in the context of system failures, rather than individual fault, it is clear that many of the failings represent a mixture of the two. Many of the actions undertaken by an individual member of the hospital staff could be analysed in terms of the *Bolam* test and be found wanting, i.e. the individual would be found to be in breach of his duty of care to the patient. But that is not the point. The systems approach suggests that we should not automatically assume that we should look for an individual to blame for an adverse outcome. What we are asking is that when an error is made, the finger should not necessarily be pointed at the doctor who made the final error. We are asking that a more considered approach be taken that looks at matters in the round, that digs a little deeper and tests the role of management and the systems that operate in the hospital.

## Failure to follow protocols (see Cases 2, 11 and 14)

The decade since the writing of *An Organisation with a Memory* has seen the introduction of numerous protocols and standard operating procedures to try to improve the service offered by the NHS to its patients: protocols for the treatment of specific diseases, to stop the spread of infections such as MRSA, for the care of outliers, for the running of Emergency Departments (ED) and

Safety Checklists for use in theatres. These can only be for the good, setting in place good working practices and, therefore, improving patient care.

A doctor can take some comfort that by adhering to a protocol he will be protected from criticism. In principle, a protocol issued by a respectable source can be regarded as a statement by a responsible body of medical opinion on what to do in a particular set of circumstances. But adherence may not always provide protection to a doctor. There may be some circumstance relevant to the individual patient that renders a particular protocol or part of a protocol inappropriate. A protocol should not replace good judgement.

## Inadequate communication (see Cases 2, 3 and 34)

Several of the errors in the vincristine case can be categorized as communication errors. This is not surprising. Many errors in diagnosis and treatment can be traced back to inadequate communication between members of the team or teams treating the patient.

Communication can be achieved through the written or the spoken word. In the vincristine example, the doctor who was to administer the drugs and who took the afternoon off should have done a formal face-to-face verbal handover with the doctor who was in charge of the ward that afternoon. Similarly, the loss of the patient's medical records prevented the staff from comprehensively assessing his needs. Both these failings, one entailing verbal, the other written communication, denied others important information.

Although communication is omnipresent and relates to all aspects of practice, we wish to point out the following issues:

- *Telephone Advice* – Frequently physicians are required to advise other staff members over the telephone. Such advice should be recorded in the medical notes or electronically to document the episode and for the information of other treating clinicians.
- *Transfer to ICU* – Poor communication between departments often causes unwarranted delays in the transfer of patients to ICU with the attendant risk of deterioration in the patient's condition.
- *Equipment* – It is surprising how often a doctor will seek some piece of equipment and discover that it is either missing or does not function. Such lack of usable equipment causes delays in treatment. Often the cause lies in the fact that staff do not report equipment faults.
- *Safety Net* – Clear instructions should be provided to patients and their carers prior to their discharge from the ward, ED or clinic. They should be told what symptoms and signs they should look out for and be advised on when and how they should seek further advice or assistance.
- *Abnormal Results* – Abnormal test results should be communicated as fast as possible, so that appropriate investigations and treatment can be instigated.

More and more information is recorded electronically rather than on paper. There are obvious advantages to this, legibility and ease of access and storage being the obvious ones. But there are dangers. There must be a system in place to ensure that test results are seen by the relevant clinicians, that the appropriate action is taken and that this is all recorded. There will need to be plans in place, for instance, for accessing the results of a consultant's patients when that consultant is away.

It is perhaps obvious, but it is worth stating all the same: communication is only achieved when someone says or writes information in such a way that the other understands. It must be clear. When it is done well, it facilitates good treatment. It is key to the smooth running of all organizations and the NHS is no exception. Communication, communication, communication: this should be the mantra of all medical teams.

Although it is possible to criticize individuals for failures in communication, there will generally be a systems element to such failings. Good communication is fostered by good leadership, the type of leadership that encourages teamwork and an atmosphere in which all members of a team, even the most junior, can feel confident in expressing themselves.

## Poor and inadequate record-keeping (see Cases 9 and 31)

We have already alluded to the importance of good record-keeping in discussing the need for effective communication. It should be seen as a subset of good communication. In the vincristine example, a junior doctor wrote IT and IV as abbreviations for intrathecal and for intravenous. He was criticized for failing to write out the words in full. Perhaps this failure was not crucial, but perhaps if he had written the words out in full, then the fatal error would not have occurred. After all, the anaesthetist managed to confuse the route of administration of both drugs, giving the vincristine intrathecally and the methotrexate intravenously, the exact opposite of what should have been done.

On a more general note, accurate and full records are often the only way of gauging deterioration in the patient's condition, allowing the clinicians to change their treatment plans to treat the patient appropriately and to set out what the intended treatment plan is and the trigger episode for review.

## Lack of knowledge and not knowing one's limitations (see Case 11)

In the vincristine example, the anaesthetist who administered the fatal dose of the drug knew how to administer drugs intrathecally, but had no oncology experience: he had never administered chemotherapy. If he had had the appropriate knowledge, he would never have administered the vincristine into the patient's spine. This action is inexcusable on many levels. In the civil courts, it amounts to a breach of the duty of care owed to the patient. The fact that the anaesthetist was inexperienced and was probably doing his best does not provide a defence. A doctor's care is always judged by the standard of the reasonable and responsible doctor. The responsible doctor in this anaesthetist's shoes should have sought assistance or at least double-checked what was required.

The same applies to any junior doctor who is learning the ropes. If he is asked to do something or finds himself in a situation outside his range of experience, then he must seek advice or assistance from someone with the appropriate level of experience. Again, we come back to the importance of communication within the team.

Although the anaesthetist should never have administered the drugs to the patient, there is a sense in which he was put in a difficult situation by failings in the specialist centre's systems. There had been an inadequate handover by the oncology Senior Registrar and the Senior Registrar on duty was unaware that the methotrexate and the vincristine had both been delivered to the theatre. This is why the authors of *An Organisation with a Memory* stressed the importance of the systems approach in analysing errors.

Of course, in stating that the junior doctor should seek assistance, we are presupposing that he will recognize when he is out of his depth. Common sense should tell him this, but there will be occasions when his own lack of experience will not be apparent to him. Where this happens, we should look higher up the chain of management and question whether his superiors are supervising him or delegating tasks to him in an appropriate fashion.

## Poor supervision and delegation (see Case 1)

Not knowing one's limitations and poor supervision and delegation may simply be flip sides of the same coin. As we have hinted, the doctor who acts outside his range of knowledge may be put in that situation by a superior who delegates an inappropriate task to him.

Within the catalogue of errors listed in the vincristine case, there are several examples of poor supervision or poor delegation. A junior doctor took the consent for the administration of the methotrexate, but failed to take the consent for the administration of the vincristine; this task should not have been delegated to him or at least he should have been supervised by a more senior colleague. Of course, the anaesthetist himself should never have been asked to administer the drugs; he lacked the experience and it was not right that the task was delegated to him.

Poor supervision and poor delegation are classic symptoms of a system that is poorly organized and a team that is not functioning effectively. They are symptomatic of poor management at some level.

## Poor prioritization

In the vincristine example, the oncology Senior Registrar was called to the anaesthetic theatre, but found himself unable to leave the ward. He told the anaesthetist that this was a straight-forward procedure and that he should go ahead without him. In the circumstances, this proved to be a bad decision and showed poor prioritization; the Senior Registrar should either have left the ward and gone to theatre or he should have asked an experienced junior doctor in oncology or his consultant to deal with this task.

Any person in a busy job must learn to prioritize effectively and doctors are no exception. A doctor can only learn this skill through experience and by weighing up the risks involved in the various decisions that he has to make.

## Tiredness and stress: lack of resources

Prioritization may not always be that easy. In the vincristine example, the oncology Senior Registrar did not know that a mistake had been made and that both the methotrexate and vincristine had been delivered to the theatre. If he had known this, he may have acted differently. But we know that he was busy on the ward, perhaps too busy. He may well have been stressed. The fact that he was expected to be in two places at the same time suggests a lack of resources at the specialist centre. It is fair to say that there will inevitably be times in the career of a doctor, when lack of resources, stress and tiredness will stand in the way of best practice.

The introduction of the European Working Time Directive should have helped to reduce stress and tiredness, but in turn it may cause difficulties with staffing rotas. These are systems issues. The solutions will not be easy. If the problems become acute, then the doctor should raise them with the hospital Trust's management. But with only a finite pot of money available for the NHS, this may not automatically bring about the desired improvement.

## Psychological factors

Psychological factors play an important role in many clinical errors. We have already mentioned tiredness and stress and these and other psychological issues will be mentioned elsewhere, but only in passing. We do not intend to provide an in-depth discussion of the psychology of error. We leave that for others to do. Our emphasis is on the case studies and what they reveal about what doctors should look for when diagnosing and treating their patients (if the reader wishes to read about the psychology of error, then we would recommend Professor Charles Vincent's *Patient Safety*, 2005).

That said, we cannot escape the psychological aspects of clinical error. We give one example to illustrate the importance of this issue: another vincristine case that ended with a fatal outcome.

A locum doctor was asked to administer vincristine to a patient out of hours. He had not administered the drug previously and the mother of the patient was on hand, watching. She had watched doctors administer the treatment several times before and knew the procedure well. She saw that the doctor was making a mistake and told him that the clear fluid (the vincristine) should be put into the vein and the yellow fluid (the methotrexate) should be put into the spine. The doctor ignored her, despite her comments, and administered the vincristine intra-thecally. Several days later the patient died.

At this point in time, this doctor lacked humility. He thought that he knew best, when he did not. If he had been prepared to listen to the mother, the patient would not have died.

### Conflicts between system issues and personal responsibility: a healthy work environment

In our Introduction, we explained that the GMC expects each doctor to fulfil his personal responsibilities. However, he may have to do this in an environment that may conflict with these responsibilities. A doctor in such a situation will be required to perform a balancing act. If that act becomes impossible, then he must 'blow the whistle' and bring the matter to the attention of his managers. Again, we repeat our mantra: communication, communication, communication. Every NHS Trust will have a Whistle Blowing Policy.

Despite the publication of *An Organisation with a Memory*, the NHS still shows symptoms of an unhealthy blame culture. The report pointed out the difficulty faced by individuals who draw attention to problems in their working environment. Its authors recommended that the NHS should foster a more open culture in which errors can be admitted without fear of discrimination or reprisal (though individuals still need to be held accountable for their actions).

We believe that the best work environments are those where good, professional teamwork comes naturally and people are pleased to come to work. There is an intangible element. It requires each person within the workplace to think about how he can help himself and others to work better together. If it can be achieved, then it should go some considerable way to meeting the aims of *An Organisation with a Memory* and the number of clinical errors should consequently be reduced.

Having looked at system errors, we now turn our attention to more specific areas of error, those that could perhaps be considered more person-centred. But before doing so, we wish to share some research that we have conducted on errors in Adult Medicine. It highlights those areas where physicians could do better as individual doctors. It has also helped us to establish the sort of errors that we need to focus on in the rest of Part 1, Section 1 and to determine the type of case studies that we should cover in Part 2.

### Evidence from the NHSLA database

The NHS Litigation Authority (NHSLA) database provides a good source of information on errors in Adult Medicine. It is important to note that the primary function for the database is as a claims management tool rather than as a source for detailed research, and any conclusions drawn must come with that caveat attached. The NHSLA is a Special Health Authority

**Table 1.1** Types of incident leading to successful litigation, 1/4/2005 to 31/3/2011, n = 1319

|  | Number | % |
| --- | --- | --- |
| Death | 422 | 32.0 |
| Unnecessary pain | 247 | 18.7 |
| Fractures | 207 | 15.7 |
| Pressure sores | 93 | 6.8 |
| Psychiatric | 31 | 2.4 |
| Bruising/extravasation | 24 | 1.8 |
| Healthcare associated infection | 14 | 1.1 |
| Brain damage | 14 | 1.1 |
| Burns | 13 | 1.0 |
| Venous thromboembolism | 9 | 0.7 |
| Anaphylaxis | 8 | 0.6 |

that manages clinical negligence, employer's liability and third party claims against NHS Trusts in England through its Clinical Negligence Scheme for Trusts (CNST) and Risk Pooling Scheme for Trusts (RPST). In the six years between April 2005 and March 2011, 1319 claims were settled in favour of the claimant in relation to the broad practice area of Adult Medicine. Many other cases will have been opened during that period and, having not yet reached a conclusion, do not feature in these figures. Indeed, some of the incidents took place as long ago as 1995/96, were inherited by the NHSLA at its inception, and took 14 years to be settled. The most common types of incident are summarized in Table 1.1.

The NHSLA was also able to provide a breakdown of the primary cause of the alleged errors that led to successful litigation in these cases. These are summarized in Table 1.2.

The damages awarded in each of the cases (excluding legal costs) ranged from £200 to £2.5m (mean £39 291). The total damages awarded over this six-year timeframe – in relation to adult medicine – amounted to £52m, with an additional £33m in legal costs.

Not surprisingly, the study shows that the commonest cause of errors lie in a failure or a delay in diagnosis and treatment. Prescribing errors also come high up the list.

Most errors in clinical practice result in little or no harm. However, the NHSLA data show that the commonest outcome in the cases analysed was death. Looking a little further down that list, unnecessary pain, fractures and pressure sores feature prominently. It is likely that some of these fractures occurred following inpatient falls.

The physical and psychological consequences to the patient and his family of these adverse incidents can be very severe. The financial cost to the NHS, especially in this age of budgetary pressure, is considerable. The largest claims resulted from cases that had led to brain damage and paraplegia. NHS Trusts

**Table 1.2** Primary cause of incidents leading to successful litigation 1/4/2005 to 31/3/2011, n = 1319

|  | Number | % |
| --- | --- | --- |
| Delayed/failed diagnosis | 281 | 21.3 |
| Delayed/failed treatment | 280 | 21.2 |
| Inadequate nursing care | 211 | 16.0 |
| Medication error | 105 | 8.0 |
| Lack of assistance/care | 60 | 4.5 |
| Failure to recognize a complication | 39 | 3.0 |
| Failure to supervise | 38 | 2.9 |
| Inappropriate treatment | 35 | 2.7 |
| Infection | 33 | 2.5 |
| Wrong diagnosis | 20 | 1.5 |
| Failure of infection control policy | 13 | 1.0 |
| Failure to interpret X-ray | 11 | 0.8 |
| Inappropriate discharge | 8 | 0.6 |
| Assault (staff) | 4 | 0.3 |
| Assault (other patient) | 4 | 0.3 |

do not pay the compensation to patients directly. They make monthly subscription payments to CNST that are calculated on their claims history, size of Trust and type of clinical specialities in the Trust. If a Trust can demonstrate that it meets specified NHSLA standards it can obtain a discount in its CNST subscription payments (at level 1, 2 or 3 – 10%, 20% or 30% respectively).

Pulling all this research together, we believe that there are certain key areas where doctors would benefit from advice. We aim to provide such advice in the following sections. This will include advice on making the correct diagnosis promptly, avoiding prescribing errors, checking test results and acting on abnormal findings, avoiding errors in practical procedures, supervising or coordinating care and discharging patients effectively. We shall start by looking at the patient consultation and how to identify the sick patient.

## The patient consultation

The patient consultation is, in a very practical sense, at the heart of the doctor–patient relationship. It gives an opportunity for face-to-face communication and for the doctor to build up a rapport with the patient and to win his trust. If it is handled correctly, at the end of the consultation, the doctor should be armed with the information that he needs to reach a diagnosis or at least to start considering differential diagnoses. And of all consultations, it is the first that is perhaps the most important; that first consultation will strongly influence all that follows. How should it be conducted?

A good medical history is essential in making a correct diagnosis. The medical history on its own is said to lead to the diagnosis in over half of all cases. Once a patient has given his account of his presenting complaint, the doctor should ask questions to clarify his understanding of the complaint and the patient's symptoms. All this is perhaps obvious, but it all comes down to communication. Good communication should aid diagnosis; poor communication will hamper it. Thus a doctor must listen carefully to patients and their carers. In the words of Sir William Osler, Regius Professor of Medicine in Oxford in the early twentieth century, 'Listen to the patient. He is telling you the diagnosis.' This requires skill and patience and can be difficult if time is short.

Doctors often see patients who speak poor English. Where this gets in the way of understanding, the doctor should find a translator who can speak the mother tongue of the patient. If a translator is not on site, most hospitals have telephone access to translators 24 hours a day. A judge is unlikely to excuse a mistake caused by a failure to find and use a translator.

After the medical history comes the patient examination. If the examination is a limited one, the doctor should make that clear in the patient's notes together with the reason why.

Once the medical history and patient examination have been completed, it is important to make a diagnosis or to consider the differential diagnoses in order of probability. The doctor should list the investigations required to clarify the diagnosis and to provide further details about the illness. A management plan should then be constructed. Following this pathway encourages a doctor to rigorously analyse the ailment afflicting the patient.

The medical history, patient examination, diagnosis, investigations and management plan should be clearly documented. It is also very important to note negative findings in the medical history and patient examination. The investigation results should be obtained and documented promptly. The importance of clear and thorough documentation cannot be overemphasized.

The requirement in the NHS to see all patients who present to the ED within four hours can sometimes cause doctors to prioritize patients inappropriately. Thus a doctor may find himself rushing the medical history and patient examination in order to meet this deadline. Errors may occur as a result. But it is no defence for a doctor to argue this in court. This, along with factors such as the stress, tiredness and depression, are issues which may adversely affect the outcome of the patient consultation. If the doctor has concerns about the systems in place at his hospital, he should discuss them with his superiors.

A delay or failure in making a diagnosis and a delay or failure of treatment are the two commonest causes of errors. The reasons behind these delays and failures are many; they include poor training, a lack of knowledge, failure to recognize when help is required and a more senior opinion is needed, and an inadequate hospital Trust and departmental induction to the job.

Hospital Trust protocols and national protocols on different conditions provide information on the symptoms that need to be asked about, the signs that need to be checked, the differential diagnoses in a given set of circumstances and the appropriate treatment plan. Likewise, various courses such as the Advanced Life Support Course or the ALERT (Acute Life threatening Events – Recognition and Treatment) Course provide very useful training in important areas of Adult Medicine, encouraging doctors to make use of standardized procedures, particularly at times of stress and urgency.

## Failure to identify a sick patient

It is easy to identify a severely unwell patient. The challenge is to spot the patient who is not yet severely unwell but who may deteriorate rapidly if he does not receive the right treatment. Such patients present alongside hundreds of other patients with self-limiting conditions.

Where a sick patient is not identified, this is usually because early warning signs of a critical illness were missed or ignored. Therefore, when an essential physiological parameter (heart rate, blood pressure, respiratory rate, $SaO_2$ or GCS) is abnormal, this needs to be carefully explored to see if it is a sign of an impending deterioration.

When cases involving sick patients who were not correctly identified are reviewed, it is often found that the patient had a single abnormal parameter and that this was not acted upon. All too often, the journey to cardiovascular shock is evident in retrospect from looking at observation charts with blood pressure falling and heart rate increasing in tandem. Reviewers generally conclude that the doctor did not act on this finding because:

- he attributed the abnormal parameter to some cause other than illness e.g. the doctor considered that the patient's tachycardia was caused by anxiety; or
- he chose to ignore a single abnormal parameter because everything else was normal; or
- he failed to recognize that the parameter was abnormal.

To try and prevent these common mistakes, various Early Warning Scores (EWS) were developed. These provide a range of defined triggers for review by a clinician and escalation where required.

On occasion, a patient can re-present to the ED critically ill after attending the ED for the first time just a few days earlier. It is natural to assume that 'something was missed' at the first attendance. In many cases this is true, but it is also true that patients can deteriorate suddenly and rapidly. While all such cases should be explored to see if lessons can be learned, it can equally be that sometimes, when patients are seen very early in the course of a critical illness, there are no early warning signs of a severe illness to identify.

This only serves to reinforce the need to give patients clear 'safety net' advice, when they are discharged from medical care: that is advice about when they should re-attend the ED or the GP, if the patient fails to get better. Such advice should be given no matter how trivial the presenting complaint may appear to be.

## Inability to competently perform practical procedures

The phrase 'Practice and Planning Prevents Poor Performance' is often used in military basic training and could be equally applied to medical procedures. Assiduously following the simple guidance below should help avoid errors whilst carrying out practical procedures.

Practical procedures require good communication skills, manual dexterity, patience, a calm and gentle touch, and supervised practice. The doctor should be aware of the limits of his competence and should not exceed them without experienced supervision (GMC – Good Medical Practice, sections 3 and 12).

The use of an assistant is also important in many scenarios. The objective should be to perform the correct procedure on the correct patient, on the correct side, competently and with appropriate consent. Plan the procedure where possible, and give adequate analgesia or sedation, in an appropriate environment.

Prepare the trolley and instrument pack. Watch a good scrub nurse at work – a doctor can learn much from a scrub nurse about safe and ergonomic methods of preparing his own kit. Ensure all the necessary instruments are present. Keep sharp instruments, needles and blades inside a tray to reduce the risk of a needlestick injury. Keep a count of needles and swabs.

Ensure that the patient is adequately monitored. An assistant should take primary responsibility for the safety and comfort of the patient whilst the doctor performs the procedure. If indicated, the doctor should check that life support equipment is present and working, and that he knows how to use it if necessary.

Good aseptic technique reduces the chance of infective complications. Empower the assistant to notice lapses and tell him to point out if gloves or instruments become contaminated.

Prevent the external surfaces of cannulae and catheters from becoming contaminated with cotton wool fibres – these can cause thrombosis if inadvertently inserted into blood vessels.

A doctor should ensure that he understands the anatomy of the procedure, and use instruments for the purposes for which they were designed. Practise using the instruments. Most commonly-used instruments are designed to be used by a right-handed operator and may not work optimally if used left-handed. Read the product inserts and instructions, especially if using a new type of catheter. Thin-walled catheters may become cracked if manipulated with metallic instruments. Examine distance markers carefully. The doctor should ensure that he knows what length of a tube or catheter will protrude from the patient at the end of the procedure.

At the end of the procedure, document the process carefully, retaining a note of the batch number and catheter type inserted. Obtain radiological confirmation of line positions if needed, record the findings and take remedial action if necessary.

Remember to talk to the patient at the end of the procedure. The doctor should explain what he has done, what should happen next, and make patients aware of potential complications.

## Failure to check test results or act on abnormal findings

It is stating the obvious to say that if tests are requested, the results have to be looked at (ideally by the doctor who ordered them). They have to be considered with the care to be expected of a competent doctor.

Life at the coalface is always more complicated. Circumstances may intervene: the doctor who actually requested the test may finish his shift before the results are available, leaving another doctor to deal with them. The handover to that doctor may have been inadequate. Alternatively, he may simply be too busy to give them proper attention, with the result that an abnormality is overlooked. While those circumstances might point to weaknesses in the system, they do not absolve the responsible doctor (or his employing hospital Trust) from a charge of negligence.

That is why it is so important that clear notes are made, pointing out the need to follow up the results of investigations.

When it comes to interpreting the results, however, the situation is different. A misinterpretation obviously might be negligent: the inexperienced doctor may not appreciate the significance of an abnormal finding, or the incompetent doctor may realize it but just not act on it. However, a competent doctor is allowed to make errors of judgement without necessarily being labelled negligent. So, in a subtle case, with confusing symptoms and signs, an independent expert may take the view that the notional competent doctor might well have made the same mistake as the one accused of negligence.

Another, not uncommon scenario is a fluctuating situation where an abnormal result comes and goes. At the time, a considered judgement may be made to 'watch and wait'. Later, with the benefit of hindsight, an independent expert may be able to pinpoint exactly when that policy ceased to be appropriate, with a clarity which was unavailable at the time, but that is with the benefit of hindsight.

## Prescribing errors

Prescribing errors are very common. The EQUIP study (2009), a prospective observational analysis of hospital prescribing showed that in the UK prescribing errors are made in disturbingly high numbers. 8.4% of prescriptions written by FY1 doctors contain errors and this increases to 10.3% amongst FY2 doctors. Consultants do slightly better but still get it wrong in 5.9% of prescriptions. Although many of these errors are minor and most are picked up in checking processes (usually by pharmacists), 1.74% of all prescribing errors are potentially lethal. If you think about the millions of prescriptions written every day in the UK, it is easy to see that in absolute terms the scale of the problem is immense.

A doctor should always refer to The British National Formulary or approved local guidelines when prescribing a medication unless he is fully familiar with the medicine, dose, route, side effects, interactions, duration of therapy and indication. Doctors should be aware that the responsibility for a mistake lies with the person who has signed the prescription. The following principles should be adhered to when prescribing medication:

- Write prescriptions legibly, ideally in capitals.
- The generic names of drugs should be used whenever possible.
- Beware of drugs with similar sounding names or which look similar when written down.
- Always double check the prescription. This is particularly important when using unfamiliar drugs, or familiar drugs in an unfamiliar setting. If calculations are involved, try to get a medical or nursing colleague to check the arithmetic. If someone questions the prescription, the prescription should be checked carefully. During working hours a pharmacist may be available to check the prescription.
- The strength or quantity to be contained in tablets or liquids should be stated (e.g. 125 mg/5ml).
- Dose frequency, and also specific times, should be stated and in the case of drugs to be taken 'as required' a minimum dose interval should be specified.
- Great care needs to be taken with the decimal point. The unnecessary use of decimal points should be avoided (e.g. 5 mg, not 5.0 mg). The zero should be written in front of the decimal point where there is no other figure (e.g. 0.5 mg, not .5 mg). To avoid confusion over the placing of decimal points, amounts less than 1 milligram should be prescribed in micrograms (e.g. 500 micrograms, not 0.5 mg).
- The correct units should always be used. Avoid abbreviations. In particular, do not abbreviate the terms micrograms and nanograms.
- The term 'Units' should always be spelt out in full when prescribing (e.g. insulin or heparin) in order to reduce the chance of 'U' being interpreted as '0' leading to a tenfold error.
- Ensure that the correct route of administration has been specified. See, for example, the vincristine example above, when the chemotherapy was administered intrathecally instead of intravenously.
- Clear plans should be in place for the necessary monitoring of drugs. For example, gentamicin levels.
- Ask about allergies, and the nature of the reaction. Document the reply that the patient has given.
- Careful consideration should be given to the information that is provided to patients concerning side effects. Some doctors believe that it is only necessary to tell patients of risks that have more than a 1% chance of occurring (the Electronic Medicines Compendium quantifies the incidence

of side effects of many drugs). This is not an accurate reflection of the law. A doctor should always consider what would be reasonable to tell the patient. For example, in many circumstances it is right to mention rare but potentially serious side effects.

- Doctors should ensure that the medication is not contraindicated. For example, beta blockers in asthma. Changes in pathophysiology are important. A drug which was appropriate at one stage in an illness may not be as the disease progresses. For example, metformin may be the drug of choice for a Type 2 diabetic early in their disease, but some years down the line when glomerular filtration rate has fallen it may become more hazardous.
- The doctor should ensure that potential interactions with other medicines that the patient is taking are identified and warn the patient about possible interactions with over the counter medicines. Where interactions may be anticipated dosage alteration may often be needed and close monitoring is obligatory. Some combinations should never be used (for example azathiaprine and allopurinol).
- Repeat prescriptions should be regularly reviewed to ensure that they are still necessary.
- The administration of medicines should be carefully documented to ensure that drugs are not given twice.
- Mistakes in the calculation and conversion of doses of opiates are a common serious prescription error. So, too, are errors in the prescription of anticonvulsants, calcium channel antagonists and antibiotics. In time, computer packages and online prescribing should become available and facilitate the correct calculation of drug doses, help with drug interactions and diminish the incidence of medication errors. However, the first error-prone element of the prescription process – a doctor making an active decision that a prescription is indeed necessary – will not be directly affected by this technology. Safe prescribing modules are part of the undergraduate curriculum and are also incorporated into several Foundation year training programmes.

## Sources of error in the case of vulnerable adults

### Failure to recognize vulnerability and abuse

Vulnerable adults do not necessarily come with a label. They may not be small in stature or physically weak. A large number of adults, some of them with learning difficulties or cognitive impairment, are vulnerable. It is imperative that all professionals involved in patient care maintain a high index of suspicion with regards to the signs and symptoms of abuse, and an open enquiring mind with respect to the risk factors associated with abuse. Paediatricians are now well versed in identifying the victims of abuse. In adult medicine, we are perhaps too quick to explain away the possible signs of abuse and to be reassured about a patient's home environment and care. Rather than being reassured, we should always seek solid evidence (assurance) of well-being and good care, triangulating different streams of information where appropriate. All NHS Trusts have a Vulnerable Adult Lead who can be contacted for advice.

## Failure to act

If a doctor has a gut feeling that something is not right, he should act on it. Action might involve consulting with seniors, involving social services or obtaining information from other sources. The care of the vulnerable adult operates in a protective jurisdiction. That is to say, professionals can and must act upon suspicion or concern, rather than requiring absolute proof. False alarms are sadly necessary if the majority of true cases of abuse are to be uncovered and tackled.

## Failure to document

During the course of a patient's involvement with the health services, a number of professionals may experience their own fleeting moment of questioning or doubt as to a vulnerable individual's safety. Unless those professionals communicate with one another effectively and appropriately, the true nature of the patient's situation may never be realized. It is imperative that the multidisciplinary team including social services and primary care is brought in to the conversation.

## Common pitfalls

- Not being suspicious enough when things don't add up – 'Think the unthinkable.'
- Failure to recognize the impact of alcohol abuse in the household.
- Failure to put the vulnerable patient's needs first. The best interests of a vulnerable patient and his relatives or carers normally go hand in hand but when there is any suspicion of maltreatment the patient's interests are paramount, above those of the carer.
- Not referring upwards at an early stage.
- Sloppy or inadequate history.
- Not admitting a vulnerable patient to hospital when abuse has not been excluded and it is not clear that home is a safe place.
- Not discussing with other agencies.
- Not checking if the patient is on a vulnerable adult register.
- Poor communication between doctors, social workers and police – 'not speaking the same language'. Doctors may often think that they have fully explained the medical findings, but actually these may not have been clearly understood by non-health professionals.
- Not documenting all discussions including telephone calls with other agencies.

- Being drawn by social workers or the police to give a definitive opinion on the cause or age of injuries when this is not possible.

## References and further reading

Department of Health (2000) An Organisation with a Memory, the report of an expert group on learning from adverse events in the NHS, chaired by the Chief Medical Officer (2000). http://www.dh.gov.uk/en/Publicationsandstatistics/Publications/PublicationsPolicyAndGuidance/DH_4065083

Dornan T, Ashcroft D, Heathfield H, *et al.* (2009) An in depth investigation into causes of prescribing errors by foundation trainees in relation to their medical education. EQUIP study. Available at http://www.gmc-uk.org/FINAL_Report_prevalence_and_causes_of_prescribing_errors.pdf_28935150.pdf

GMC (2008) *Consent: Patients and Doctors Making Decisions Together.*

GMC (2009) Good Medical Practice. www.gmc-uk.org/guidance/good_medical_practice.asp

Hampton JR, Harrison MJG, Mitchell JRA *et al.* (1975) Relative contribution of history taking, physical examination and laboratory investigation to diagnosis and management of medical outpatients. *BMJ* 2: 486–9.

Markert RJ, Haist SA, Hillson SD *et al.* (2004) Comparative value of clinical information in making a diagnosis. *MedGenMed* 6(2): 64.

Office of the Public Guardian, Department of Health and Welsh Assembly Government (2005) Mental Capacity Act 2005 – Summary. http://www.dh.gov.uk/prod_consum_dh/groups/dh_digitalassets/documents/digitalasset/dh_080403.pdf

Reynard J, Reynolds J, Stevenson P (2009) *Practical Patient Safety.* Oxford University Press.

Vincent C (2005) *Patient Safety.* Churchill Livingstone.

# Section 2: Medico-legal aspects

## Error in a legal context

So far, we have discussed medical error in general, nonlegal terms. Now we shall consider it from a strictly legal point of view. We shall look at issues surrounding consent and confidentiality. In a legal context, as soon as one mentions error, the word negligence immediately surfaces.

If a doctor makes a mistake in the treatment of a patient, then he or his family, may decide to pursue the hospital Trust (or the doctor himself, if he provided the treatment in a private capacity) for compensation. Generally speaking, in order to win compensation, the patient will have to prove that the Trust's doctor employee was negligent. It is important to remember that negligence as a legal concept is all about financial compensation and that the law has defined negligence in specific terms. Not all errors will be considered negligent.

## Negligence

Before looking in detail at what is relevant to this book, clinical negligence, we need to know the basics that lie behind what is called the tort of negligence (tort is simply the old French word for wrong. In modern legal terms, it forms a branch of legal study).

In principle, a person is liable in negligence if he has breached a duty of care owed by him to another in such a way as to cause damage to that person. What does this mean? In practical terms, in order to decide whether an act or omission is negligent, a lawyer must break this formula down, looking at each of its constituent parts, phrase by phrase, word by word. For example, he will ask himself whether a duty of care exists between the injured person and the alleged defendant.

It may not always be clear whether a duty exists in a given set of circumstances, but as far as medical treatment is concerned, it is assumed that a doctor owes such a duty of care to his patient. The key questions in any clinical negligence case are whether that duty of care has been breached and then if it has, whether any damage has been caused as a direct result of that breach.

*Avoiding Errors in Adult Medicine*, First Edition. Ian P. Reckless, D. John M. Reynolds, Sally Newman, Joseph E. Raine, Kate Williams and Jonathan Bonser.
© 2013 John Wiley & Sons, Ltd. Published 2013 by John Wiley & Sons, Ltd.

## Clinical negligence

### Has there been a breach of duty?

When the treatment of a patient comes under scrutiny in a potential clinical negligence claim, the first question that will be asked is: was that treatment in accordance with the standard of a body of reasonable or responsible physicians? If it was, then the private doctor or the NHS Trust will not have breached their duty of care; but if the treatment does not accord with the standards of a reasonable body of physicians, then they will have breached that duty.

This test was first formulated by the House of Lords in the case of *Bolam v Friern Hospital Management Committee* in 1957. Hence the *Bolam* test.

Over the years, a body of legal case law has built up that indicates how this *Bolam* test should be applied. How, for instance, should we look on a case, where in a given set of circumstances, one set of physicians may treat a patient in a certain fashion, while others would adopt a different approach? In case law, so long as both bodies of physicians are reasonable or responsible, then it would not matter which one of the two approaches the doctor adopted. In other words, it is possible to have more than one correct approach to treatment.

But this begs the question: who determines whether you have breached your duty of care?

When an NHS Trust receives a Letter of Claim from solicitors representing a patient or family, it is likely that to obtain ongoing funding the patient or family will have investigated the case and gone to medical experts who have written reports critical of the care provided. On first inspection, there is a case for the Trust to answer.

In response, the lawyers for the Trust will instruct experts to look at the allegations made against it. The experts will be asked to consider both breach of duty and causation. So in the first instance, the answer to the question is that the opinions of the independent medical experts, as interpreted by the lawyers, will determine the progress of the case. If both experts, the expert for the family and the expert for the Trust believe that the care was substandard (i.e. care did not accord with the standards of a reasonable body of physicians), then it is likely that the Trust will concede, with the prior authority of the NHSLA, that the treating Trust doctors and, therefore, the Trust according to the principle of vicarious liability (since the doctors are Trust employees), has breached the duty of care to the patient. But what happens, if the expert for the Trust concludes that the treating clinicians have not breached their duty of care?

At this point one may say that the difference in the two opinions, that of the family's expert and that of the Trust's expert, simply reflects two different approaches. Have we not just said that a doctor will not breach his duty of care, so long as he acts in accordance with a reasonable body of opinion? Has not the Trust's expert supported the clinician's care? Is this not enough?

The short answer is that it may be, but not necessarily so.

The *Bolam* test has been qualified, or rather refined, by the case of *Bolitho v City and Hackney Health Authority*. The judges in this 1993 case stated that although one group of so called 'reasonable practitioners' may adopt a certain approach to treatment, if that approach does not stand up to logical analysis, then a doctor cannot expect his treatment of the patient to be endorsed, if he adopted that apparently 'reasonable', but illogical approach to treatment. This is just one way in which the competing views of experts may be resolved. But it may come down to something less tangible: merely that one expert is more believable and persuasive than another.

At the end of the day, if the case cannot be determined by other means, it will come before a judge, who will hear all the evidence, listen to the experts and decide which of them is more persuasive. It is, of course, the judge who will be the final arbiter. But before then, evidence will be disclosed, meetings will be held and views will crystallize. The experts for the opposing sides will have met and their opinions may shift one way or the other. The reality is that few cases will go before a judge. They will either be settled out of court or the patient or family will decide to drop the case. Doctors need to understand that an NHS Trust, when authorized by the NHSLA may settle out of court without accepting liability – often simply because the costs associated with even a successful defence may be unacceptably high. As public authorities the Trust and the NHSLA have a duty to ensure that public funds are used to best effect with an ongoing costs/benefits analysis of chances of success.

## Causation

Let us assume that the patient or family prove that the doctor or Trust has breached their duty of care to the patient. This does not automatically mean that the patient will be awarded any damages. In order to obtain compensation, they must clear the causation hurdle. They must demonstrate that on the balance of probability the breach of duty was the direct cause of some injury or damage.

In some cases, causation is uncomplicated and straightforward. In others, it can be fiendishly complex. In the context of this book, we shall not delve too deeply into its intricacies, but hope to give you some idea of the basic concepts.

As an example of straightforward causation, take the case of an elderly man with COPD and a left sided pleural effusion. The doctor places a chest drain, but too low and on the wrong side. He performs the procedure without ultrasound and damages the patient's liver. The patient loses a large amount of blood and suffers a cardiac arrest. The patient is resuscitated but has clear cognitive problems. The family will easily prove causation: the poor performance of the procedure has caused the patient's injury.

Causation will be far less easy to prove in a case of septicaemia. A student is admitted to the Emergency Department with a rash which the doctor should have diagnosed as signifying meningococcal septicaemia. Within a matter of hours, the patient's condition deteriorates and she dies on ITU the next day. The causation question to address is: would the patient's life have been saved if appropriate antibiotics and fluids had been administered, when she presented? This question may prove difficult to resolve. Its answer will depend on a careful analysis by the experts of the medical and nursing notes to see how the patient's condition deteriorated during her time in hospital and a judgement on how effective earlier treatment would have been.

## Damages

The purpose of a claim in negligence is to provide the patient or family with compensation for any harm done to him through substandard care. Once it is established that the Trust has breached its duty of care to the patient and that that breach has caused injury, the court will move on to determine how much should be awarded in damages.

Clearly, it is impossible to adequately compensate someone in monetary terms for the physical disabilities they may suffer as a result of negligence, but the idea behind compensation is to put the patient in the same position as he would have been in, if the error had not been made.

The patient will be awarded a sum of money which is designed to compensate him for his pain and suffering and loss of amenity. He will also receive a sum to compensate him for any monetary expense arising directly from the negligence which he has incurred in the past and will incur in the future: for example, the costs of physiotherapy, travel costs and future care.

Finally, he will be compensated for the future losses that he will incur as a result of the negligence. The sorts of loss will depend on the severity of the patient's injury and an assessment of the patient's life expectancy and likely future earning potential in the absence of the injury. In the most severe cases of brain damage, the compensation for future loss could include sums for loss of earnings, the cost of buying and adapting a suitable home, the costs of nursing care, physiotherapy, occupational therapy, speech therapy and computer technology to aid in communication. Over the lifetime of a young brain damaged patient the loss that he will suffer as a result of negligence could easily be several million pounds, depending on his life expectancy. Ongoing financial commitments (for example, the care and support of any dependent children) will also be assessed in relation to the amount of any damages awarded. The patient may receive the damages as a one-off lump sum payment. Alternatively, he may receive periodical payments spread over his lifetime.

If a patient dies as a result of negligence, then his or her estate and dependants may be awarded a sum for pain and suffering, funeral expenses and a sum representing the patient's financial and non-financial input into the family. The patient's husband or wife would also receive statutory bereavement damages that are presently fixed at £11 800.

Ironically, if the patient dies with no dependants, then the damages could very limited, just a few thousand pounds.

## The limitation period

An adult injured through medical negligence has three years to start his claim formally in the courts. (This three year period runs essentially from the time when the negligence occurred, but is more accurately defined by when the person harmed knew of the negligence). Although the court can extend this limitation period in certain circumstances, if he fails to start court proceedings within these three years, he can no longer pursue his claim.

However, if a person lacks mental capacity, the limitation clock may never start to run. He can then bring a case at any point in his life. 'Mental capacity' in this context means the ability to run one's own financial affairs; it is different from the test for capacity in consent cases (see below).

When a patient dies, his personal representatives will have three years to start proceedings. This three-year period runs from the date of death or when it was known that there had been a mistake, if this is later.

## Jurisdictions

The United Kingdom is divided into a number of different legal jurisdictions. In certain areas of law, England and Wales, Scotland and Northern Ireland have their own, different set of rules, as do also the Channel Islands and the Isle of Man. However, what we have said above about clinical negligence applies to all jurisdictions. (The Scottish word for tort is delict, but the principles are the same.) However, these jurisdictions do have their own rules for procedures that affect how a case is litigated.

The defence of the NHS trusts in clinical negligence cases is also organized in different ways. Thus the NHSLA is responsible for cases in England, whereas Welsh Health Legal Services is responsible in Wales. In essence, however, defence of such cases is financed out of central funds, no matter where in the United Kingdom NHS hospital cases are litigated.

## Issues around consent

Consent to treatment is the foundation of patient autonomy and is fundamental to the trust that should exist between the doctor/nurse and the patient. It is required for all aspects of treatment, from the administration of routine antibiotics to the most complicated and demanding of surgical procedures.

From the standpoint of the physician confronted with an ill patient to treat, his wish is to help that patient by applying his medical knowledge to cure and alleviate suffering. That said, the general rule is that a patient, no matter what his age, a child or adult, cannot be made to accept treatment that he does not want. It is does not matter how painless, beneficial and risk-free that treatment would be; the patient is fully within his rights to refuse what he is offered. It is irrelevant that the consequences of refusal may be dire or fatal.

To put it bluntly, in legal terms, if the doctor treats without the patient's consent, he is liable in the tort of battery. In layman's terms, he commits an assault.

That is the general rule. But there are exceptions to this rule which will be discussed below. But we must first describe the framework within which consent operates.

## Validity of consent

A patient's consent is valid, if it is given voluntarily, if the patient has the mental capacity to understand the nature of the treatment and he has been given sufficient information about the procedure to understand its nature. In the context of errors, we are, therefore, interested in failures on the part of the physician to provide sufficient information and failures to respect the autonomy of the patient, i.e. ignoring his wishes. Before looking at these error types, we wish to focus on the issue of capacity to consent.

## Capacity

The law considers an adult to be someone who is aged 18 or over. Children aged 16 and over are presumed to have the same capacity as an adult to consent to medical treatment (Family Law Reform Act 1969 and Mental Capacity Act).

A child under the age of 16 may have capacity, provided he is capable of understanding the nature of the proposed course of treatment and is capable of expressing that wish. Such a child is referred to as *Fraser* competent. There is no fixed age at which a child becomes *Fraser* competent.

However, a doctor should not assume that just because a patient is over 16, he is competent to consent: the patient may lack capacity and the doctor will need to assess whether the patient has capacity, by applying the general rules for competency. A person is competent, if he can:

- understand and retain information pertinent to the decision about his care, i.e. the nature, purpose and possible consequences of the proposed investigations or treatment, as well as the consequences of not having treatment;
- use this information to consider whether or not he should consent to the intervention offered;
- communicate his wishes.

Sometimes, the very condition from which the patient is suffering may affect their ability to make decisions about the treatment of their condition and deny them the capacity to make effective treatment decisions. Take the hypothetical case of a patient with anorexia nervosa, who refuses treatment for her condition. Although she has the capacity to consent to treatment, the courts may doubt whether she had sufficient understanding to refuse treatment, because it is a feature of anorexia nervosa that patients have a distorted view of what is a normal body image and this renders them incapable of making an informed decision. In circumstances such as this, a doctor should contact the Trust's solicitors for advice and, if appropriate, make an application to the court for directions on what treatment, if any, is to be provided in the patient's best interests.

## Devolving responsibility for consent to another

In paediatric practice, someone with 'parental responsibility' or a natural parent must give consent, where the child lacks competence. There is no equivalent for patients over the age of 16 except where a Lasting Power of Attorney, with the relevant clauses, has been activated.

## Mental Capacity Act and Lasting Power of Attorney

The Mental Capacity Act 2005 came into effect on 1 October 2007. It provides a much clearer legal framework for decision making in relation to those who lack capacity to direct those decisions with autonomy. Prior to the inception of the Act, the legal framework for decision making in this context was drawn from a variety of individual rulings (Case Law).

The Act aims to empower and protect people who may lack capacity on an ongoing basis to make some decisions for themselves, for example, some people with dementia, learning disabilities, mental health problems, stroke or head injuries. Alternatively, a lack of capacity may arise because at the time an urgent decision needs to be made, an individual temporarily has impaired consciousness whether due to an accident or being under anaesthetic, or his ability to make a decision may be affected by the influence of alcohol or drugs.

The Act makes it clear who can take decisions in which situations and how they should go about this. It enables people to plan ahead for a time when they may lack capacity. The Act covers major decisions about someone's property and affairs, healthcare treatment and where the person lives, as well as everyday decisions about personal care (such as what someone eats), where the person lacks capacity to make the decisions themselves.

There are five key principles:
- a presumption of capacity;
- individuals being supported to make their own decisions;
- individuals are entitled to make what others might regard as unwise decisions;
- a decision made under the Act must be made in their best interests; and
- any decision made should represent the least restrictive option in respect of their basic rights and freedoms.

The Act also makes provisions on the subject of restraint. Restraint is only permitted if the person using it reasonably believes it is necessary to prevent harm to the person who lacks capacity, and if the restraint used is a proportionate response to the likelihood and seriousness of the harm.

The Act describes two situations where a designated decision-maker can act on behalf of someone who lacks capacity:

- Lasting Powers of Attorney (LPAs) – The Act allows a person to appoint an Attorney to act on his behalf if he should lose capacity in the future. In addition to managing decisions relating to property and affairs, the Act also allows people to empower an Attorney to make health and welfare decisions. Issues relating to property and affairs were also covered by Enduring Powers of Attorney (EPA) which the LPA replaces. Before it can be used, an LPA must be registered with the Office of the Public Guardian.
- Court appointed Deputies – Deputies can be appointed to take decisions on welfare, healthcare and financial matters as authorized by the Court of Protection. They are not able to refuse consent to life-sustaining treatment. They are only appointed if the court cannot make a one-off decision to resolve the issue.

In order to administer the powers and functions described above, a new Court of Protection has been created which has jurisdiction relating to the whole Act. The court can make declarations, decisions and orders affecting people who lack capacity and make decisions for, or appoint Deputies to make decisions on behalf of, people lacking capacity.

A Public Guardian who has several duties under the Act has also been created. The Public Guardian and his staff is the registering authority for LPAs and Deputies. He supervises deputies appointed by the court and provides information to help the court make decisions. He works together with other agencies, such as the police and social services, to respond to any concerns raised about the way in which an Attorney or Deputy is operating.

The Act makes several other important provisions:

- It creates the role of Independent Mental Capacity Advocate (IMCA) who is instructed to support a person who lacks capacity and has no one to speak for him, such as family or friends. They have to be involved where decisions are being made about serious medical treatment or a change in the person's accommodation where it is provided, or arranged, by the National Health Service or a local authority, and may be involved in abuse cases. The IMCA makes representations about the person's wishes, feelings, beliefs and values and brings all relevant information to the attention of the decision maker. The IMCA can challenge the decision-maker on behalf of the person lacking capacity if necessary.
- It enshrines in Law the ability of individuals to make Advance Decisions to refuse treatment. The Act sets out the two important safeguards of validity and applicability in relation to Advance Decisions. An Advance Decision

must be in writing, signed and witnessed. In addition, there must be an express statement that the decision stands 'even if life is at risk' which must also be in writing, signed and witnessed.

- The Act introduces the criminal offence of ill treatment or wilful neglect of a person who lacks capacity. A person found guilty of such an offence may be liable to imprisonment for a term of up to five years.
- The Act describes clear principles that should be applied in relation to the involvement of those who lack capacity in medical research.

### Respecting patient autonomy

As a rule, a patient or his Attorney have the right to refuse treatment for any reason whatsoever. However, this general rule does have exceptions.

## An attorney refusing treatment

Attorneys must exercise their power to give or withhold consent for the treatment of the patient in his best interests, not their own. They may withhold consent for any number of reasons. If the patient suffers from a terminal condition, they may decide that he would not benefit from further painful treatment which only has a slim chance of prolonging life. Whether that decision is the right one must be judged from the standpoint of what is best for the patient.

So what happens, when an attorney for whatever reason refuses the treatment suggested for the patient against the doctor's advice? If it is confronted with this situation, through the Trust's solicitors, the Trust should apply to the Court for an opinion. In making its decision, the Court will look at the best interests of the patient; his welfare will be of paramount concern. If this scenario arises on a doctor's watch, then he should contact the Trust's solicitors immediately. They may be able to make an application to the Court and obtain a decision within a matter of hours if necessary in an urgent situation. In the meantime, treatment may proceed according to the treating doctor's perception of best interests if it is urgent and cannot be deferred.

## A patient without capacity refusing treatment

A competent adult can refuse any treatment for himself, no matter how vital. Where the patient is not judged competent, treatment can proceed if it is in his best interests. However, it is best practice for such decisions to be taken in conjunction with the patient's family and carers (as advocates) or in the absence of such, an Independent Mental Capacity Advocate (IMCA). The capacity of the patient and the need to involve advocates will vary according to the nature of the proposed intervention, its urgency and the consequences of not undertaking the intervention.

## Emergency treatment

In an emergency, a doctor will be within his rights to treat a patient in his best interests if he lacks capacity to consent. Such treatment is justified by the legal doctrine of necessity as restated in the Act.

## Information to be provided

Consent to treatment should be an expression of patient choice. But if a doctor does not give the patient sufficient relevant information concerning the proposed treatment, then the choice he makes will not be properly informed. This will invalidate any 'consent' or agreement to treatment and lay the doctor open to legal criticism and a potential claim. Such an error will surface, as far as the law is concerned, when the treatment for which 'consent' was given ends in a poor outcome. It is at that point that a patient or family could raise concerns about the consent process.

In terms of the information to be given, a doctor's duty is defined by the terms of the *Bolam* test for negligence. In other words, he is to give the information regarding risks, side effects and consequences that is thought appropriate in the circumstances by a reasonable or responsible body of fellow physicians. Doctors commonly think that there is no need to warn of risks that have a less than 1% chance of occurring. In some cases, this may be good practical advice as a rule of thumb, but it is not an accurate reflection of the law. A doctor should always assess the individual patient and the condition in order to gauge what information they require and identify any patient specific risks, for example impaired eye sight in one eye prior to procedure. In such a case, rather than just quoting the procedure specific risks, the risks for the individual patient are greater as he already has impaired eyesight in one eye should there be adverse outcome.

The decision as to what risks a doctor should mention depends on a balancing of the benefits of the procedure and the risks. One matter that is of concern to clinicians generally is that if they advise of all the risks, then this will unnecessarily discourage their patients from undergoing procedures. Whether this is a valid consideration will depend on the circumstances of the case. If a procedure carries a less than 1% chance of paralysis, it may still be advisable to warn of this risk if the operation is designed to alleviate a slight discomfort. But there may be no need to warn patients of this small risk if the operation is an urgent life-saving procedure.

On a more practical level, a clinician should try to explain the nature of the procedure or treatment, the effect of no treatment and what other treatment options are available in terms that the layman can understand. He must attempt to communicate effectively. That does not mean to say that he will necessarily be successful.

Nowadays, many surgical procedures come supported by lengthy booklets and videos explaining the nature of the operation, its purpose and its risks.

Judges have commented, however, that such booklets seem to be drafted in order to prevent litigation rather than from a desire properly to inform the patient. It is certainly true that these booklets in themselves do not prove that the patient has given valid consent. The treating clinician must still discuss the procedure with the patient and his advocates to ensure that they sufficiently understand its nature, purpose, benefit and risks.

Similarly, just because patients have signed a consent form saying that they understand the operation and its risks, it does not necessarily mean that they have received adequate information. At best a signature is only an indication that consent may have been given. In England, Department of Health guidance requires that the national Consent to Treatment Forms are completed and signed by the patient and doctor prior to a treatment where the patient will be under general anaesthetic. Consent to minor procedures or tests does not always need written consent. A patient's consent for minor procedures not requiring a general anaesthetic can be implied from the actions of a patient. So if a patient holds out his arm for an injection, the doctor can infer that he has given his consent for the injection to be administered.

As a general comment, the issue of consent is a complex area of law. The GMC has published guidance in the form of a booklet entitled 'Consent: Patients and Doctors Making Decisions Together'. The actual process for obtaining patient consent can itself often be the basis of a legal claim. If the recommended DOH consent process is not followed it can lead to allegations of failure to obtain informed consent and failure to advise the patient of the associated risks.

## Deprivation of Liberty Safeguards

The provisions of the Mental Capacity Act 2005 include the Deprivation of Liberty Safeguards (DOLS) that focus on vulnerable people within society who, for their own safety and in their best interests, may need to be accommodated under care and treatment regimes for which they lack the capacity to consent. Such regimes may have the effect of depriving them of their liberty.

Under DOLS, the Managing Authority (a care home or an NHS Trust) must apply to the Supervisory Body (the Local Authority or PCT respectively) for authorization of Deprivation of Liberty (Standard Authorization). The Managing Authority can award itself authority to deprive an individual of liberty for up to seven days if the need is urgent and where Standard Authorization has been applied for but not yet granted.

The Supervisory Body commissions a series of best interest and medical assessments and either grants or refuses authorization. The standardized assessments are carried out by specifically trained health or social care professionals (Best Interests Assessors), who cannot be directly involved in the care of the patient, and specially trained doctors with expertise in mental health (Medical Assessors), who can know the patient.

## Confidentiality

'Whatever I see or hear, professionally or privately, which ought not to be divulged, I will keep secret and tell no one': these words are those of Hippocrates. They form part of his oath and are still an important element of the doctor/patient relationship. Hippocrates simply gives voice to the fact that a full history is an essential requirement for diagnosis and treatment and the patient must feel able to tell his doctor everything relevant to his condition, even the most embarrassing and personal details, without fear that those details will be divulged to others. Updating the words of Hippocrates and putting them in legal terms, a doctor owes a duty of confidentiality regarding information about his patient or others acquired in his capacity as a doctor. This duty applies whether the information comes from other people or from the patient himself.

If a doctor breaches this duty of confidentiality, then he could be sued for damages, but more likely he will be reported to the GMC. As far as it affects clinicians, the law concerning confidentiality is fashioned from a number of different sources. Primarily, there is the common law duty of confidence (constructed from court judgements). In the last few decades, this has been supplemented by a number of Acts of Parliament: namely, The Access to Health Records Act (1990), The Data Protection Act (1998) and The Human Rights Act (1998). These different elements combine to create a more or less coherent whole. What we have set out below represents an outline of this legal framework.

Starting with the basics, a doctor can disclose information to others, if he has the patient's consent. But consent can be implied. Most patients understand that a doctor will share information about them with other members of the healthcare team. In other words, the doctor can assume that he has the patient's implied consent to do this.

This may seem obvious, but a doctor should, where appropriate, consider just how far this implied consent extends for any given course of treatment. It may not extend to highly personal details about the patient that he has learned in treating some other, previous illness. The doctor in charge of the team should consider what information it is necessary to disclose, when treating the patient. If he discloses information of a highly personal nature to the members of his team, then he should make it clear that the information is disclosed to them in confidence. He should also tell the patient and/or the family that the information has been shared with other members of the team.

## Disclosure without consent

There are a number of circumstances in which a doctor can legitimately disclose patient information to another without the consent of the patient:
- Abuse or neglect: Where the doctor believes that the patient may be the victim of abuse or neglect and the patient is unable to give or withhold

consent for disclosure, then the patient's health is of paramount importance and he may disclose his belief to an appropriate, responsible person.
- Statutory obligation: A doctor is required to notify the appropriate authorities, if he attends upon someone suffering from certain infectious diseases, or known or suspected to be addicted to controlled drugs.
- Public interest: A doctor may disclose patient information, if he believes that the patient presents a real risk of danger or serious harm to the public. For example, a patient who is thought or known to be driving a motor vehicle whilst prohibited from doing so through ill health. Likewise, if a doctor believes that a patient's mental instability could manifest itself in extreme violence to others, then he may disclose this belief to the proper authorities.
- When ordered by the court to do so: A doctor should not assume that simply because a lawyer or some figure of authority, such as a police officer, asks for disclosure of the patient's records, they are entitled to see the medical records. He should only disclose the records, if the patient has consented or the court has ordered disclosure and a copy of the written court order has been supplied.

## Caldicott Guardians

Each NHS Trust should employ a Caldicott Guardian. His role is to ensure that patient information is dealt with in an appropriate fashion and that there are systems in place to ensure that all clinicians and the Trust generally respect the duty of confidentiality that exists between them and the patients that they serve. Therefore, he should be a first port of call, if an issue arises concerning the use of confidential information.

Much of the work of the Caldicott Guardian relates to compliance with statutory obligations. It would be useful to take a look at some of those requirements.

## Data Protection Act 1998

Generally speaking, patients seek disclosure of their records under the Data Protection Act 1998. It is most frequently 'used' for this purpose. However, disclosure of records represents only a small part of its purpose. Most importantly it sets out rules for what it describes as the 'processing' of 'personal data': in the context of medical records and treatment, read 'use' of 'medical records and information'.

In summary, the Data Protection Act 1998 describes the principles of data protection in the following terms:
1. Personal data must be processed fairly and lawfully.
2. Personal data must be obtained only for one or more specified and lawful purpose, and should not be further processed in any manner incompatible with that purpose or those purposes. (In other words, if you are given

information about a patient, you cannot use it for purposes other than the treatment of that patient. Certain histories may make entertaining after-dinner stories, but they will not comply with the Act.)

3. Personal data must be adequate, relevant and not excessive.
4. Personal data must be accurate and, where necessary, kept up to date.
5. Personal data must not be kept for longer than is necessary. (This is a matter of discretion. It may be incorrect to keep personal information that was relevant to the treatment of one condition, if it has no relevance to a subsequent condition.)
6. Appropriate technical and organizational measures must be taken against unauthorized or unlawful processing of personal data and against accidental loss or destruction of, or damage to, personal data.
7. Personal data must not be transferred to a country or territory outside the European Economic Area unless that country or territory ensures an adequate level of protection for the rights and freedoms of data subjects (i.e. patients) in relation to the processing of personal data.

Point 6 will have the greatest impact on a doctor's day to day practice. The Trust should have in place a number of Information Governance protocols to safeguard the confidentiality of patient information. For example, the physical paper records should be carefully stored in a secure environment. Any electronic data (e.g. radiographs) should be protected with access only allowed to those with passwords.

There are any number of 'obvious' things that a doctor can do to ensure compliance, like marking letters with confidential information 'private and confidential'; avoiding the temptation to discuss patient care with colleagues whilst in public areas; taking care over typed handover sheets, making sure that they are not left in the canteen or on the bus; and not leaving computer screens on to be read by prying eyes.

### Access to Health Records Act 1990

Prior to the Data Protection Act 1998, records were disclosed to patients under the Access to Health Records Act 1990. Though this Act has now largely been superseded, it still applies to the disclosure of records, where the patient has died. Disclosure under The Access to Health Records Act 1990 is only allowed to certain, specified individuals: namely, to the personal representative of the deceased or to a person who has a civil claim arising out of the death of the patient. Care must be taken to make sure that the records are disclosed to the appropriate person. The duty of confidentiality extends beyond death.

### The Human Rights Act 1998

Article 8 of the Human Rights Act 1998 establishes a right to 'private and family life'. Applying this right to medical treatment, the patient can expect his privacy and the confidentiality of his medical records to be properly protected.

However, the Act does not grant privacy as an absolute right without limit or exception. There are occasions, when health bodies and clinicians may limit or supersede a patient's rights.

Without going into excessive detail, it is generally accepted that compliance with the Data Protection Act 1998, the common law duty of confidentiality and the common law and statutory exceptions mentioned above will satisfy the requirements of the Human Rights Act 1998.

# PART 2

# Clinical cases

## Introduction

Having set the scene with a general discussion of error and medico-legal theory, we now come to the backbone of our book: the case studies. We have chosen 34 cases that are based on the pooled experience of the authors. Most cases are not directly factual accounts. Where scenarios are based on actual cases, they have been anonymized and altered to preserve confidentiality and to maximize the educational messages of the case.

In addition to a medical and legal comment, at various points in the description of a case, we ask direct questions that are designed to engage the reader in the case and to get them to think about how they would respond if they were in that situation. The case studies conclude with key learning points.

As much as it is a science, medicine is also an art. There is often room for argument over the finer points of a case. The medical expert and legal opinions may well differ. But that does not obviate the general conclusions that we draw, or the benefits that can be gained from the reading of these case studies.

*Avoiding Errors in Adult Medicine*, First Edition. Ian P. Reckless, D. John M. Reynolds, Sally Newman, Joseph E. Raine, Kate Williams and Jonathan Bonser.
© 2013 John Wiley & Sons, Ltd. Published 2013 by John Wiley & Sons, Ltd.

# Section 1: Civil liability, negligence and compensation

# Case 1  A shaky excuse

Paul Turner is a 34-year-old self-employed painter and decorator who is normally fit and active. He has been diagnosed as having probable multiple sclerosis after a self-limiting episode of left hemi-sensory disturbance 3 years ago and, more recently, trigeminal neuralgia which has settled on treatment with carbamazepine 400mg bd.

Mr Turner presented to his GP with shortness of breath, a productive cough, vomiting and fever. The GP detected signs of right-sided basal consolidation on examination and Mr Turner looked ill. Worried about pneumonia, the GP has sent Mr Turner to the Acute Medical Unit (AMU). Mr Turner has no known allergies or drug intolerances.

## What is your initial management?

Dr Smith, the Core Medical Trainee (CT1) on the AMU agrees that Mr Turner has a history and clinical findings suggestive of pneumonia. He documents a respiratory rate of 24, a temperature of 39.4 °C, reduced percussion note at the right base and bronchial breathing. Mr Turner's blood pressure is 92/62 and he has a sinus tachycardia of 104. Chest X-ray confirms right lower lobe pneumonia.

Dr Smith calculates a CURB-65 score and decides that Mr Turner scores only 1 (for a raised urea), but he is aware that the patient looks more unwell than this score alone would suggest. He consults the hospital formulary and decides to admit Mr Turner and treat him with intravenous co-amoxiclav and oral erythromycin for the first 48 hours, along with 5 litres min$^{-1}$ oxygen, paracetamol as required, intravenous rehydration and subcutaneous dalteparin for prophylaxis against venous thromboembolism. The Consultant Physician on take agrees with the management plan.

After 48 hours Mr Turner is generally better – his temperature has settled, he is less hypoxic and is no longer requiring supplemental oxygen. He remains lethargic and feels shaky. The intravenous cannula is removed and he continues on oral antibiotics with a plan for 7 days in total and discharge home the next day. However, on the morning of discharge the nurses report that Mr Turner is unsteady on his feet and the Ward FY1 doctor notes that he has mild truncal ataxia and a tremor. The junior doctor is concerned that Mr Turner is developing a further episode of demyelination.

## What would you do now?

The FY1 telephones the on-call registrar and asks specifically about the management of an acute brainstem demyelinating episode. Without seeing the patient, the registrar suggests an MRI scan should be requested and this is scheduled for the next day. In the meantime, Mr Turner appears to be recovering well from his pneumonia but he feels nauseated, lethargic and his cerebellar signs are deteriorating. The MRI is performed the next day but is not reported until late in the afternoon – there is no clear evidence of any change compared with a previous scan performed 14 months ago and specifically there is no new cerebellar or brainstem lesion. An opinion is requested from neurology and the neurology SpR agrees to see Mr Turner the next afternoon if he can be brought down to outpatients.

## What is your diagnosis?

When seen the next day by the trainee neurologist, Mr Turner is drowsy, has a marked tremor, nystagmus in all directions of gaze and is so ataxic he cannot stand. He is vomiting intermittently and feels awful. The neurology SpR is concerned about acute demyelination but also raises the possibility of an acute cerebellar syndrome associated with mycoplasma infection.

At this stage the Ward Pharmacist returns from leave and writes on the patient's drug chart that care needs to be taken when erythromycin is co-prescribed with carbamazepine but does not contact and speak to the medical team directly.

*Avoiding Errors in Adult Medicine*, First Edition. Ian P. Reckless, D. John M. Reynolds, Sally Newman, Joseph E. Raine, Kate Williams and Jonathan Bonser.
© 2013 John Wiley & Sons, Ltd. Published 2013 by John Wiley & Sons, Ltd.

By day 6, Mr Turner is worse and the neurology SpR decides to discuss the case with her consultant. The next morning while waiting to hear back from neurology, the consultant physician does a ward round and is very concerned about Mr Turner's drowsiness and notes there is now new onset confusion. The drug chart is reviewed and the Ward Pharmacist's comments are revealed. An urgent carbamazepine plasma concentration is requested and 3 hours later the laboratory confirms that Mr Turner has carbamazepine toxicity.

The FY1 crosses off the erythromycin from the drug chart and asks the nurses not to give the carbamazepine until it has been reviewed at 48 hours. He tells Mr Turner that he has 'had a reaction to one of the tablets' and that things should now improve. This is indeed the case and after a further 72h in hospital Mr Turner is well enough to go home. However, he still feels washed out and it takes another week before he can contemplate returning to work.

Some months later he attends his GP practice for treatment of an infected hand wound and the GP asks is Mr Turner is allergic to any antibiotics. Mr Turner says he is not sure but something happened to make him very unwell during the recent admission and so the GP checks the discharge summary and reveals that Mr Turner developed carbamazepine toxicity caused by co-administration of erythromycin. Mr Turner is angry and feels he was misled and that the treatment provided in hospital delayed his return to work. He writes a letter of complaint to the hospital asserting negligence and demanding recompense for loss of earnings and inconvenience.

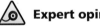 **Expert opinion**

The initial clinical assessment was appropriate and although Dr Smith deviated from the strict letter of local guidance on antibiotic usage, it was reasonable to do so given the concern that Mr Turner was more unwell than the CURB-65 score suggested.

The use of erythromycin was debatable but the BTS guidelines do allow for its use in community acquired pneumonia. However, Dr Smith was unaware of the potential interaction with carbamazepine and did not check for possible drug interactions.

Macrolide antibiotics (and erythromycin in particular) are subject to a significant number of drug interactions because of their inhibitory effects on CYP3A4 and P glycoprotein. No doctor can be expected to remember all drug interactions and so it is essential to check (usually by referring to the interactions section of the British National Formulary (BNF)), especially when using combinations of drugs with which one is unfamiliar. Electronic prescribing will flag up potential interactions but experience with some systems shows that prescribers become fatigued by constant reminders and alerts and either mentally switch off or in fact disable software which triggers them. Remember – when you write a prescription, even if you are simply transcribing it and did not initiate therapy in the first place, you are responsible for ensuring that the details are correct and for checking interactions and incompatibilities.

The management of Mr Turner was left in the hands of junior staff between the post take ward round and day 7 – this is unacceptable and may well have contributed to the delay in diagnosis of carbamazepine toxicity.

The ward pharmacist was away but as soon as she returned she flagged up the possible interaction but failed to talk to anyone or appreciate the significance of Mr Turner's new symptoms. Over-reliance on safety nets (like a pharmacist checking a drug chart for interactions) may reduce self-reliance and experience, and creates greater risk when the safety net fails or is absent.

Failing to give a full and accurate explanation of what has gone wrong is unacceptable. This was an example of poor prescribing practice and the consequent iatrogenic illness was entirely avoidable.

## Legal comment

The letter of complaint should be responded to with a factual explanation of events. There is no scope for legal compensation under the formal NHS complaints process, although reimbursement of expenses and *ex-gratia* payments are permitted with no admission of liability.

The Department of Health guidance does permit a parallel investigation of a complaint and a potential clinical negligence claim, provided the complaint investigation and response does not prejudice a Trust's ability to defend a future clinical negligence claim. This should be discussed between the Trust's complaints manager and legal manager.

The use of the word 'negligence' and request for 'reimbursement' would indicate the likelihood of a future clinical negligence claim. If the patient wishes to pursue a claim for compensation either as a litigant in person or with the assistance of a claimant clinical negligence solicitor, the allegations will need to be reported by the Trust's legal department to the NHS Litigation Authority (NHSLA) so that insurance reserve figures can be placed on the potential claim and an investigation of liability can take place.

Under the Clinical Negligence Pre-action Protocol, the healthcare records would need to be disclosed to the claimant, reviewed by the Trust's legal department and comments obtained from Trust staff involved in the patient's care to enable the Trust/NHSLA to provide a Letter of Response to the allegations within 4 months of receipt of the Letter of Claim.

In English civil tort law, an assessment is made as to whether, on the balance of probability a healthcare professional of similar seniority and speciality would have acted in the same way; or whether the care provided fell below that reasonably expected by the 'responsible body of professional opinion'. Compensation would only be forthcoming if there has been a breach of duty of care and this had directly caused physical or psychiatric harm to the patient.

Although no individual practitioner can be expected to remember all drug interactions, they have a duty of care whenever they write up a new drug to make reasonable efforts to identify any potential problems. The interaction between macrolide antibiotics and carbamazepine is very well described and is clearly flagged up in the BNF. Failure to check for potential drug interactions and hence to take precautionary measures is a common problem.

The lack of senior clinical input between the post take ward round and the business round a week later does not represent a good level of care and might well influence the outcome of a negligence claim.

Organizational Learning is an important aspect of clinical governance. The clinical events described should have triggered an Incident Report Form to be completed by Trust staff for review by the Trust's clinical risk team. Whilst there were no long term sequelae for this patient, the near miss should have prompted reporting and underlined the need to improve communication between pharmacy and medical team, and the need to escalate unexpected changes in the condition of a patient to senior clinical staff.

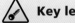 **Key learning points**

### Specific to the case
• The interaction between macrolide antibiotics and carbamazepine is very well described and is clearly flagged up in the BNF. Progressive ataxia and sedation should have raised the suspicion of carbamazepine toxicity but the team involved did not look beyond the patient's previous history of demyelination and were unable to change their thinking when evidence before them indicated they were incorrect.
• Adverse drug reactions and drug interactions are extremely common and account for 6.5% of all acute hospital admissions.

### General points
• All prescribers have a duty of care whenever they write up a new drug to make reasonable efforts to identify any potential problems. Failure to check for potential drug interactions and hence to take precautionary measures is a common problem.
• The lack of senior input between the post take ward round and the business round a week later does not represent a good level of care and might well influence the outcome of a negligence claim.
• The on call registrar was too ready to provide an opinion without seeing the patient and by so doing was probably unaware of the co-prescription of carbamazepine and a macrolide.
• Organizational learning is an important aspect of clinical governance. The clinical events described should have triggered an Incident Report Form to be completed by Trust staff for review by the Trust's clinical risk team.

## References and further reading

British National Formulary (http://www.bnf.org) (last accessed 18 March 2012).

British Thoracic Society. Updated (2009) BTS guidelines on management of community acquired pneumonia in adults. *Thorax* 64 (Suppl 3): iii1–iii55

Lim W, Eerden M van der, Laing R *et al.* (2003) Defining community acquired pneumonia severity on presentation to hospital: an international derivation and validation study. *Thorax* 58(5): 377–82.

Pirmohamed M, James S, Meakin S *et al.* (2004) Adverse drug reactions as cause of admission to hospital: prospective analysis of 18 820 patients. *BMJ* 329:15–19.

Richards D, Coleman J, Reynolds J, Aronson J (2011) *Oxford Handbook of Practical Drug Therapy.* Oxford University Press, 2nd Edition.

# ⚠ Case 2 Making matters worse

Mrs Turnbull is a 74-year-old lady with moderate COPD having smoked 10 cigarettes per day for over 50 years. Six years ago, she had two episodes of pulmonary oedema associated with paroxysmal atrial fibrillation. When she was in sinus rhythm she had a reasonable exercise tolerance and echocardiography showed mildly impaired left ventricular function, left atrial dilatation (6.5 cm) and moderate mitral regurgitation. Both episodes of atrial fibrillation had occurred despite concurrent beta blocker therapy.

## What therapeutic options were available to Mrs Turnbull's physician six years ago?

In view of her poor tolerance of rhythm change a decision was made to commence Mrs Turnbull on amiodarone, initially at a dose of 200 mg three times a day, reducing to twice a day after a week, and after a further week coming down to 200 mg once a day as maintenance therapy. The consultant cardiologist who saw her in outpatients wrote down these instructions for Mrs Turnbull and also wrote a clear letter to her general practitioner. A one month follow-up appointment had been made but for some reason this did not occur and Mrs Turnbull was not reviewed in outpatients at all.

Over the next four years, Mrs Turnbull remained quite well but then she began to develop worsening shortness of breath and was troubled by a persistent cough. Mrs Turnbull's GP had been treating her for what he assumed to be progressive COPD and more recently also for probable heart failure. After a particularly bad few days she is admitted on a general medical take where she is found to be short of breath at rest, apyrexial, and hypoxic with a PaO2 of 7.9KPa on room air. There are fine inspiratory crepitations to both mid zones, the JVP is not seen and there is a pan systolic murmur at the apex. Mrs Turnbull is seen by Dr Wagstaff, a core medical trainee.

## What treatment should Dr Wagstaff institute?

Dr Wagstaff agrees with the likely diagnosis of heart failure and requests a chest X-ray. The chest film is consistent with heart failure but it also raises the possibility of pulmonary fibrosis. After several days treatment for heart failure with no real improvement a high resolution CT scan is performed which shows widespread mid and lower zone pulmonary fibrosis consistent with amiodarone-induced pulmonary toxicity.

The amiodarone is withdrawn and Mrs Turnbull is commenced on oral steroids but her breathlessness progresses. After a protracted and difficult few weeks in hospital, she dies. Her family ask why she was put on such a dangerous medication in the first place and why she was not warned of possible side effects. They also question why she was not monitored and ask whether the adverse impact of amiodarone could have been spotted earlier, and been reversed.

## How should Dr Wagstaff reply?

## ◎ Expert opinion

Paroxysmal atrial fibrillation can be difficult to control and if a patient has not responded to beta blockade and tolerates the arrhythmia poorly, then amiodarone, although associated with serious side effects, is a reasonable treatment to consider. However, close monitoring is necessary and generally one would expect to do baseline tests including: chest examination (or chest X-ray), ECG, liver and thyroid function tests. These should be repeated six monthly thereafter. If a patient achieves suppression of the paroxysmal atrial fibrillation then a dosage reduction to 100 mg a day may be justified.

Patients should be informed of the likelihood of side effects (about 50% of patients will develop side

*Avoiding Errors in Adult Medicine*, First Edition. Ian P. Reckless, D. John M. Reynolds, Sally Newman, Joseph E. Raine, Kate Williams and Jonathan Bonser.
© 2013 John Wiley & Sons, Ltd. Published 2013 by John Wiley & Sons, Ltd.

effects on long-term therapy though generally only about 20% will need to stop the amiodarone). Careful monitoring will detect significant thyroid disease and six-monthly chest examination or X-ray may alert the prescriber to the development of pulmonary disease in time to avert irreversible damage. The presence of pre-existing pulmonary pathology probably increases the risk of pulmonary fibrosis. It also may delay recognition of the true cause of any reduction in exercise capacity.

If serious pulmonary side effects do arise then withdrawal of amiodarone may be associated with improvement or cessation in progression. If a chest X-ray had been done it is likely that Mrs Turnbull's fibrosis would have been picked up sooner allowing prompt withdrawal of the amiodarone and she might not have gone on to develop irreversible disease.

The family have asked if this might have been spotted sooner and the simple answer has to be yes. There was a clear failure of adequate communication between the cardiologist and the GP. It is commonplace for a 'shared care protocol' to be drawn up to cover the use of drugs like amiodarone in which the responsibilities of the specialist and the GP are clearly set out. In particular responsibility for undertaking monitoring and determining any dosage adjustments should be stipulated at the outset. No such shared care arrangement was in place for Mrs Turnbull and the GP was inexperienced in the use of amiodarone and did not appreciate the risk or the need for long term monitoring.

The following is an example of a typical shared care protocol:

Shared care assumes communication between the specialist, GP and patient. The intention to share care should be explained to the patient and accepted by them. Patients should be under regular follow-up which provides an opportunity to discuss drug therapy.

(a)  Hospital Consultant
  ○  Carry out ECG monitoring, serum potassium measurements, LFTs and TFTs prior to treatment and communicate to patient's GP.
  ○  Initiate treatment as per the local hospital protocol and prescribe until the dose is stable (normally first 3 weeks) and/or the GP formally agrees to shared care.
  ○  Write to the GP requesting shared care and outline shared care protocol criteria.
  ○  Liaise with GP regarding changes in disease management, drug dose, missed clinic appointments.
  ○  Ensure clinical supervision of the patient is undertaken by follow-up as appropriate.
  ○  Ensure the patient understands the nature and complications of drug therapy and their role in reporting adverse effects promptly.
  ○  Be available to give advice to GP and patient.
(b)  GP
  ○  Prescribe amiodarone once the dose is stable.
  ○  Carry out ECG monitoring (where appropriate), serum potassium measurements, chest examination, LFTs and TFTs every six months and communicate to patient's consultant.
  ○  Advise the hospital consultant of any clinical changes where appropriate.
  ○  Monitor for adverse effects as detailed above.
(c)  Patient
  ○  Report any adverse effects to their GP and/or consultant.
  ○  Have regular monitoring as outlined above.
  (Extract of Amiodarone Shared Care Protocol reproduced with kind permission from Area Prescribing Committee, Oxfordshire 2011)

## ⚠ Legal comment

As a core medical trainee, Dr Wagstaff, may not be the most appropriate member of the team to have the discussion with the family. Under the NHS 'Being Open' policy, the consultant in charge of Mrs Turnbull's care should facilitate a factual explanation and discussion. It is not entirely clear at this point in time whether or not Mrs Turnbull's family plan to take any legal action against the Trust or the GP. In any event, an early personal statement of regret or apology would not be seen as a formal admission of liability.

The incident event occurred some four years ago. The Trust's retrospective investigation into what happened and what information was communicated between primary and secondary care may be hampered by the passage of time. Such an investigation should take place within a formal process such as the NHS complaints process or in accordance with the Trust's incident reporting guidelines. Any investigation should be undertaken in the knowledge of the GP (and a notification should be made to the relevant Primary Care Trust which has a responsibility for clinical governance).

Although the key event occurred many years ago, the date of knowledge for the family and Mrs Turnbull's estate is only recent. In the circumstances, at the discretion of the complaints manager, the recent date of knowledge may permit an investigation of a complaint if the consultant cardiologist and other staff involved in arranging follow-up outpatient appointments still work for the Trust and there has been no loss of organizational knowledge. It would be important to understand the organizational arrangements for a cardiology outpatient appointment four years ago and to understand what the shared care protocol arrangements were at that time.

Mrs Turnbull's family may decide to bring legal action against the Trust and/or GP. The Limitation Act 1980 requires that legal proceedings must be commenced either within three years from the date of the death or within three years from the date of knowledge. Although the episode of care was over four years ago, the claim may not be statute barred if a judge is persuaded that the date of knowledge for the family of an adverse event is later and there are no insurmountable evidential barriers to prejudice the defence of a claim by the Trust.

From the expert opinion it is likely, on the balance of probability, that if there had been better communication and documentation between the consultant cardiologist and GP that Mrs Turnbull would have received a one month follow-up appointment and had ongoing monitoring. The reasons for the failure to follow-up are unclear but, on the balance of probability, if Trust staff omitted to follow their departmental procedures for follow-up of this type of patient, the Trust would be held liable, subject to expert evidence, that regular monitoring would have led to withdrawal of amiodarone and altered the patient's outcome.

Damages of a modest amount would be awarded to Mrs Turnbull's estate under the Law Reform (Miscellaneous Provisions) Act 1934 (LRA), based on the losses for which Mrs Turnbull could have claimed at the instance before her death. The following heads of damages may be appropriate. In the case of a lingering death (e.g. a protracted death as a result of disease), the amount of the award for pain and suffering, and 'loss of amenity' will depend upon the actual level of pain and the time for which the pain is experienced. Although the estate is entitled to claim lost net earnings, since Mrs Turnbull was retired at the time of her death, no claim could be made for loss of income. Reasonable funeral expenses are specifically provided for in section 1(2)(C) of the LRA 1934. If a relative has been caring for Mrs Turnbull up to the time of her death, the expenses incurred by the relative in visiting Mrs Turnbull in hospital or supplying for her needs will be recoverable. Dependents of the deceased who suffer financial loss as a result of a person's death may also claim for loss of dependency, statutory bereavement award and funeral expenses under the Fatal Accidents Act 1976.

## ⚠ Key learning points

### Specific to the case
- Need for clear shared care protocol when prescribing amiodarone.
- Do not assume deteriorating respiratory symptoms are simply explained by pre-existing disease (COPD).

### General points
- Hospital specialists have a responsibility to ensure follow up and monitoring occur and should not assume the GP will be expert in the use of a drug which may seem commonplace in hospital practice.
- A GP should not take on responsibility for prescribing a drug without understanding the need for monitoring and putting the appropriate arrangements in place.
- Legal proceedings must commence within three years of the date of an adverse incident or within three years of the date of knowledge for that event.

# Case 3 Chase the bloods

Mrs Chung is a 59-year-old woman who has come to the emergency department because she feels very weak, is dizzy and at times has pins and needles in her hands. She reports that the weakness has been a gradually progressive problem over the last five days. Normally she is a very active lady who works long hours in her family business and her only past medical history is of oesophageal reflux and mild hypertension for which she takes omeprazole 20 mg a day and bendroflumethiazide 2.5 mg. She is anxious and the emergency department FY2 doctor who sees her thinks she is probably hyperventilating but asks the medical registrar on call to see her at 15.20 that afternoon.

## What other diagnoses should be considered at this stage?

There is little to find on examination other than the observation that Mrs Chung does indeed appear weak and is unable to get out of bed without assistance. The medical team arrange some blood tests which show she has a sodium of 133 mmol/l, potassium of 2.9 mmol/l and a creatinine of 63 mmol/l. A diagnosis of weakness due to hypokalaemia is made and the bendroflumethiazide is discontinued.

## Was this a reasonable assumption?

Mrs Chung is given intravenous saline with 40 mmol/l potassium and she is commenced on oral potassium replacement therapy and she is reassured and told she can probably go home the next morning if the repeat blood tests are better. Further investigations have been sent including an adjusted calcium which is phoned back by the laboratory later that evening to the ward – it is 1.2 mmol/l. The staff nurse informs Dr Briggs, the on call house officer, who assumes this is an ionized (rather than an adjusted) calcium and takes no further action.

## What should Dr Briggs have done?

Late the next morning the admitting team review Mrs Chung and are pleased to see that her potassium is now 3.5 mmol/l and they decide to send her home. Just before she goes the calcium result is noted and it is assumed that an error, perhaps of transcription, has occurred.

## If it is believed an error has been made, is it reasonable to simply repeat the test?

A repeat blood test is sent at midday but the team are busy and no one looks out for it later that afternoon and so Mrs Chung goes home as arranged at 17.00. The result was on the laboratory computer by 13.30 (the repeat value is still 1.2 mmol/l and the laboratory have also done a magnesium which is reported as < 0.1 mmol/l) but the day team missed it and the evening team have not been alerted to the fact that these results are outstanding and so no action is taken.

The next day the medical registrar who admitted Mrs Chung sees the result but as these values are 'lower than I have ever seen before – probably taken from the drip arm' she rings Mrs Chung's GP and asks if another sample can be sent just to be sure. When the practice nurse rings Mrs Chung that afternoon, she is answered by her husband who is very distressed and says his wife has just collapsed with a seizure. The ambulance is called and Mrs Chung is found to be in ventricular fibrillation. A prolonged resuscitation attempt ensues and she is brought back to hospital where she is given intravenous calcium and magnesium and makes a slow and difficult recovery. She has irreversible brain injury as a result of the circulatory arrest and although she eventually is able to go home she is unable to contribute to running the business and needs prompting and help with even the most basic tasks.

*Avoiding Errors in Adult Medicine*, First Edition. Ian P. Reckless, D. John M. Reynolds, Sally Newman, Joseph E. Raine, Kate Williams and Jonathan Bonser.
© 2013 John Wiley & Sons, Ltd. Published 2013 by John Wiley & Sons, Ltd.

## ⚛ Expert opinion

Mrs Chung has a rare but well documented complication of her proton pump inhibitor therapy – hypomagnesaemic hypoparathyroidism, and it is perhaps not altogether surprising that this was not recognized at the outset. However the family make a claim against the hospital based on the fact that the cardiac arrest was preventable and that the results of investigations showing the dangerously low calcium level were available on the evening she was admitted but no appropriate action was taken. The delay in recognizing the problem was compounded by inadequate handover arrangements and the erroneous assumption that the calcium and magnesium concentrations were too low to be credible and must have been artefactual.

If an error is suspected an incident form should have been completed and the test result confirmed or refuted with the minimum of delay. In fact it would have been very quick and easy to check the calcium level on the blood gas analyser in the Emergency Department without waiting for formal laboratory estimation. When an investigation is requested it is the responsibility of the person(s) making the request to look out for and act as necessary on the result. With frequent shift changes, handover arrangements are crucial.

A related situation occurs with emergency chest X-rays which are likely to be seen and interpreted by non-radiologists during an emergency admission and a formal radiological report may not follow for some days, by which time the patient may well be 'off the radar' and have gone home. Incidental radiological findings unrelated to the initial presentation may well have been missed by a non-expert reporter (e.g. a small but suspicious nodule behind the first rib) and although a report exists, if no one is looking out for it then the next time it is read may be months later when the patient presents with an inoperable lung tumour. Safety nets must be put in place to ensure that abnormal findings are flagged up appropriately and are dealt with. It is not acceptable to assume that your responsibility automatically goes as you walk out of the hospital.

## ⚖ Legal comment

Assessment of liability with regard to breach of duty seems clear cut: individual human errors, caused by incorrect assumptions and by systems factors have resulted in Mrs Chung being discharged prematurely. The results of low calcium were known to Trust employees and if these test results had been recognized and acted on then, on the balance of probability, the cardiac arrest could have been prevented.

This is likely to be a high value quantum case with significant compensation awarded; both in terms of the extent of Mrs Chung's ongoing care needs but also the loss of her value to the family business.

Mrs Chung has irreversible brain injury as a result of circulatory arrest. The family's lawyers will need to submit evidence about the loss of income for the family business: for example, will the business now need to employ an extra person to do Mrs Chung's work and has there been a reduction in profit and increase in outgoings as a result of her inability to work? Until what age would Mrs Chung ordinarily have been expecting to work? There will be quite considerable care requirements for Mrs Chung with assistance with personal care, activities of daily living and mobility. Independent expert reports will be required from nursing care, occupational therapy, and physiotherapy experts. Her family will have to consider adaptations to their current residential accommodation (or a possible move if this is unsuitable for the care requirements of Mrs Chung) for which they will also need to obtain expert evidence.

In some legal cases, where liability is fairly clear-cut, an early admission of liability by the NHSLA will result in judgment being entered and the focus of the legal case becomes the assessment of damages, i.e. quantum settlement. On the basis of an admission of liability, the patient's solicitors will sometimes apply for an interim payment – so as to assist the family in the interim with essential and pressing care needs – rather than waiting for the final damages settlement.

## 🔑 Key learning points

### Specific to the case
• Responsibility for following up and acting upon test results lies with the requesting clinician unless responsibility has been formally transferred through a handover or a standard operating protocol employed by the department.

### General points
• Once liability is admitted, settlement is determined on the basis of multiple factors including costs incurred by the victim of the medical error (for example, need for nursing care) and earnings missed as a result of injury.
• Early admission of liability allows for an interim payment to be made whilst full assessment of damages calculation take place.

# Case 4 Falling asleep en-route

Mr Aziz is a 68-year-old man who has been brought to the Emergency Department by ambulance. He had been referred to the on-call medical team by his GP with a 48-hour history of cough and increased shortness of breath. The ambulance staff diverted to the Emergency Department en-route as he had deteriorated in the vehicle.

Dr Singh, a staff grade doctor, reviews Mr Aziz and finds him to be flushed and pyrexial (38.3 °C). He is barely responsive, grunting incomprehensibly to painful stimulus.

## What other information do you want to know?

Observations show a blood pressure of 156/92 and a regular pulse of 96. The respiratory rate is 8 per minute and the pulse oximeter registers 86%. Mr Aziz's medication list, which was brought in by the ambulance staff, includes salmeterol, tiotropium and theophylline. Dr Singh notes that oxygen is being administered via a non-rebreathe mask and questions carbon dioxide narcosis. He immediately reduces the oxygen flow to 2 litres per minute via nasal cannulae whilst undertaking an arterial blood gas analysis:

pH 7.15, $pO_2$ 8.1 kPa, $pCO_2$ 16.2 kPa

## What course of action would you advocate at this point in time?

Dr Singh's working diagnosis is one of an infective exacerbation of COPD complicated by $CO_2$ retention. Following blood tests (including blood cultures), he prescribes intravenous antibiotics, prednisolone, nebulizers and oxygen at 2 litres per minute via mask or nasal cannulae according to patient preference. Over the next twenty minutes or so, Mr Aziz's level of consciousness improves. He is transferred to the ward, via radiology.

The on-call medical team visits Mr Aziz on the ward several hours later for a routine review and finds him lying flat, unresponsive and making only occasional respiratory effort. Oxygen is being administered at 5 litres per minute via a facemask. The Consultant asks for an urgent blood gas to be carried out which shows: pH 7.08, $pO_2$ 7.0 kPa, $pCO_2$ 21.2 kPa

## What would you do now?

The team use a bag and mask in order to improve Mr Aziz's ventilation whilst awaiting assistance from the anaesthetist. During intubation, despite all appropriate precautions, he aspirates significant volumes of gastric content into his lungs. He is transferred to ITU but develops multi-organ failure over the next 48 hours. A decision is made not to offer renal replacement therapy and Mr Aziz dies four days after admission.

## What are your thoughts about Mr Aziz's overall management? How should the hospital review his care? What should his wife be told?

## Expert opinion

Although Mr Aziz's initial history was limited, there was a clear story of worsening shortness of breath and cough preceding an abrupt deterioration in the ambulance. Carbon dioxide narcosis was promptly recognized and efforts were made to treat it.

Whilst it may seem reasonable to simply reduce the inspired oxygen concentration in a closely monitored environment such as the Emergency Department, Dr Singh should have ensured that Mr Aziz was prescribed and given a known and fixed dose of oxygen via *Venturi* mask. Dr Singh should also have made efforts to obtain objective evidence of an improvement in Mr Aziz's $CO_2$ levels prior to transfer from the Emergency Department.

In addition, Dr Singh failed to handover the concern that Mr Aziz had become unwell as a direct result of

*Avoiding Errors in Adult Medicine*, First Edition. Ian P. Reckless, D. John M. Reynolds, Sally Newman, Joseph E. Raine, Kate Williams and Jonathan Bonser.
© 2013 John Wiley & Sons, Ltd. Published 2013 by John Wiley & Sons, Ltd.

giving high dose oxygen. It is not enough to make an entry in the notes or drug chart – Mr Aziz was very unwell on admission and this should have been conveyed verbally to the nursing and medical teams who took over Mr Aziz's care from ED.

Mr Aziz's care was reported to the hospital's clinical risk management team via the incident reporting system. An investigation was launched. Simultaneously, the case was discussed at the acute medicine morbidity and mortality meeting, with input from a respiratory specialist. In the event, it appears that the hospital porter inadvertently administered 5 litres of oxygen per minute when switching the oxygen supply from piped to bottled in preparation for transfer. A second porter conveyed Mr Aziz from radiology to the ward and, having not met Mr Aziz before, was not aware of the precipitous fall in his level of consciousness. On the ward, the oxygen was switched over like for like. Nursing staff assumed, given that the diagnosis of $CO_2$ retention had been made in the Emergency Department, that the appropriate oxygen therapy was being administered. No check was made against the prescription chart.

It seems that a catalogue of errors befell Mr Aziz as he passed through the healthcare system – high-dose oxygen therapy in the ambulance; recognition of the problem in the Emergency Department but an inadequate response; a simple error on the part of portering staff; inadequate supervision of oxygen therapy by nursing staff in the emergency department or on the ward; and, the absence of a face-to-face medical or nursing handover.

The attempts to revive Mr Aziz on the ward and subsequently in the intensive care unit were appropriate. The threshold for intubation and ventilation is often set rather higher than it ought to be for patients with a history of COPD. In this case, it is likely that the iatrogenic component to Mr Aziz's clinical state prompted action. There was potentially a place for noninvasive ventilation in the emergency department after Mr Aziz's conscious level had begun to improve but whist he was acidotic and retaining $CO_2$. The absence of a second blood gas estimation meant that this treatment was not given appropriate consideration.

The hospital should be open and honest with Mr Aziz's family.

## ⚠ Legal comment

The fact that a doctor acts in a suboptimal manner does not necessarily mean that the doctor has been negligent in his/her actions or omissions. The actions in this case have been within the bounds of acceptable practice but nevertheless the patient has suffered an adverse outcome.

Whilst each doctor owes a duty of care to his patient, the overarching legal liability rests with the Trust as it has vicarious liability for the actions of its employees. Hence in this scenario, although the actions of an individual employee may not necessarily have been negligent, the culmination of the patient's interaction with the healthcare system has resulted in his death. In these cases rather than investigating each element that may have contributed to the patient's death, the legal representative for the patient's estate is likely to allege 'res ipsa loquitur', that is to say, the thing speaks for itself. The solicitor would invite the court to an inference of negligence because the death of the patient is such that there can be no other explanation. It may be impossible to know what in fact transpired and in this scenario the Trust would have to produce evidence to rebut the presumption of negligence by offering a plausible, non-negligent explanation.

The legal representatives acting for the Trust would seek to argue that proper care was exercised but that regrettably the adverse outcome was extremely rare or impossible to explain in the light of current knowledge. In any event, the claimant has to still surmount the burden of proof which even where breach of duty is clear, the cause of the injury cannot be proved on the balance of probability. Moreover, the court would need to decide what would the outcome have been for this patient had care been optimal.

In relation to the aspiration at the time of intubation, one needs to consider whether this represents unnecessary harm or unavoidable risk. Doctors have a duty at all times to act in the best interests of their patients. All clinical interventions carry a degree of risk and the assessment that is undertaken by doctors on an ongoing basis is whether the benefit of the intervention is greater than the unavoidable risk of performing the procedure.

Where the care of the patient passes between different NHS organizations they are all represented by the NHS Litigation Authority. In this example the NHSLA would represent both the ambulance Trust and the acute NHS Trust. Liability would then be apportioned between the co-NHS defendants. Most often, where the NHS is admitting liability, dispute between the two NHS co-defendants is not encouraged as this may lead to wasted costs.

The action of one public authority may interrupt the chain of causation such that the impact of an NHS organization's care early on in the patient care pathway is superseded by the actions of a subsequent legal entity. This may provide the first NHS organization with a causation defence.

Where there has been an adverse incident which is properly investigated in accordance with the Trust's incident reporting policy, then in accordance with the NHS 'Being Open' policy it is most common for the report and action plan to be shared with the patient or the patient's family. The Trust needs to think about the most sensitive way of informing and maintaining communication with the patient's wife, not only providing her with a paper copy of the report but also facilitating a meeting and discussion of the contents of the report since it contains clinical vocabulary and concepts which may be unfamiliar to a lay person. It may be equally important to the patient's family that there is evidence of organizational learning and that any action plan has been completed prior to a closure of a Serious Incident Requiring Investigation (SIRI) process.

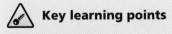 **Key learning points**

### Specific to the case
- Oxygen is a medicine and should be prescribed like any other.

### General points
- It is possible for negligence in the round to be alleged by a claimant, rather than examining each of a series of events in detail.
- The NHS Litigation Authority will represent multiple NHS organizations where liability may be distributed along a patient pathway.

# Case 5  Bad luck or bad judgement

Daphne Hardcastle is a 52-year-old publican who presents to the Emergency Department following an episode of left-sided weakness and slurred speech. Her symptoms, which lasted for approximately 40 minutes, have fully recovered upon arrival. Mrs Hardcastle's blood pressure is 168/94. Her pulse is 75 and regular. Mrs Hardcastle is a smoker and drinks approximately 40 units of alcohol per week. She is a driver and lives with her husband and three dogs. She is assessed by Dr Wilde, an FY2 doctor in the Emergency Department.

## How should Dr Wilde manage Mrs Hardcastle?

Dr Wilde makes a brief assessment of Mrs Hardcastle and establishes that there is no persisting neurology. Heart sounds are normal, blood pressure measurements remain in the region of 160 mmHg systolic and the cardiac monitor shows a regular rhythm. Capillary blood glucose is normal at 5.4 mmol/l. Dr Wilde draws bloods and sends them for routine measurements and a random total cholesterol. She calculates an ABCD$^2$ score of 4 which places Mrs Hardcastle at moderate risk of stroke in the next 48 hours. Dr Wilde faxes a referral to the TIA clinic and advises Mrs Hardcastle to report at 09.00 am the next day according to the Trust's protocol. Dr Wilde elects not to actively manage blood pressure, expecting it to be checked and followed up the next morning in clinic. Dr Wilde gives Mrs Hardcastle a single dose of aspirin 300 mg and discharges her with reassurance. She explains that Mrs Hardcastle must not drive for a month following the index event.

## Has Dr Wilde's management been appropriate? Is there anything else that you would have done?

Mrs Hardcastle's husband is awoken at around 2.30 am by loud grunting noises. Mrs Hardcastle has fallen out of bed and is lying on the floor. She is making some effort to get up but seems unable to move her right-hand side or speak. She does not seem to notice her husband as he approaches from the right to help her and appears to be drifting in and out of full consciousness. He calls an ambulance which attends within minutes. Mrs Hardcastle is blue lighted to the Emergency Department, arriving 20 minutes later.

## How should Mrs Hardcastle be managed?

Mrs Hardcastle is seen by Dr Phillips, a registrar, who makes a clinical diagnosis of a left total anterior circulation syndrome. He speaks to the acute stroke team but it is decided that the time of onset is not clear and could have occurred at any time after Mrs Hardcastle had gone to bed that evening. Hence, she is not eligible for thrombolysis. Mrs Hardcastle's blood pressure is 176/90 and an ECG reveals fast atrial fibrillation. The chest is clear. Following a failed swallow screen, Mrs Hardcastle has a nasogastric tube inserted. She is given low dose metoprolol for rate control and transferred to the stroke unit. Six hours after admission, she has a CT scan of the brain which demonstrates established infarction throughout the entire left MCA territory.

## Could Mrs Hardcastle have been managed any differently over this 24-hour period? Are there any further interventions that ought to be considered?

### Expert opinion

Mrs Hardcastle's management by Dr Wilde was generally good. An appropriate assessment was made and an evidence based risk tool was then utilized to determine further management and the urgency of specialist review. Dr Wilde would have expected Mrs Hardcastle

*Avoiding Errors in Adult Medicine*, First Edition. Ian P. Reckless, D. John M. Reynolds, Sally Newman, Joseph E. Raine, Kate Williams and Jonathan Bonser.
© 2013 John Wiley & Sons, Ltd. Published 2013 by John Wiley & Sons, Ltd.

to access brain and carotid imaging in the rapid access TIA clinic the next morning. With a blood pressure measurement in ED of 168/94, arguments could be made either way in relation to the urgency of commencing an anti-hypertensive agent. With the safety net of a clinic appointment within 24 hours and the expectation that this would be followed up, most physicians would have acted as Dr Wilde did. With the full resolution of symptoms (and a diagnosis of TIA), it is appropriate to commence aspirin prior to brain imaging. It is important to recognize however that a small proportion of patients presenting clinically with a TIA will have experienced minor intra-cerebral haemorrhage. The only criticism that can be made of Dr Wilde's management is the lack of a documented electrocardiogram. One wonders whether Mrs Hardcastle might have been in atrial flutter at the time of initial assessment which, in the context of TIA, would have led to immediate anticoagulation. However, commencing warfarin on the first attendance in ED would not conceivably have altered the outcome here.

In relation to ongoing management, Mrs Hardcastle should be urgently assessed by stroke specialists. Given her clinical state and the radiological findings, she is at high risk of malignant MCA syndrome. In this syndrome, oedema causes further damage to other areas of the brain including the ACA territory and the hindbrain. It carries mortality in excess of 50%. Mrs Hardcastle ought to be considered for neurosurgical intervention in the form of hemi-craniectomy.

## ⚠️ Legal comment

The criteria for a finding of negligence in English tort law are the existence of a duty of care, a breach of that duty of care and a foreseeable injury occurring as a result of the breach. All three elements must be fulfilled if a patient is to succeed in being entitled to compensation.

In English tort law a doctor is not deemed negligent if he/she acts in accordance with the opinion of a responsible body of medical practitioners, skilled and practised in that art. The 'Bolam' test has more recently been adjusted by the requirement that a medical opinion must also be 'reasonable' and based on evaluation of the risks and benefits associated with a particular procedure to be capable of withstanding logical analysis.

Where clinical opinion conflicts, a judge reviewing the case must assess the rationality of the two opinions. The courts recognize that professional opinion may be divided in terms of a more conservative or more interventional approach and due consideration must be given to the different modes of medical management which may apply to the same clinical specialty; even if one accepted management course is pursued only by the minority of doctors.

An adverse outcome in the course of medical treatment can be unforeseen. Despite appropriate clinical management of the patient there may be an adverse outcome. Adverse outcome is not necessarily the indication of poor/negligent care.

Where there has been an adverse outcome and there is thought to have been a breach of duty of care, there must be an established causal link with the alleged breach of duty in order to prove negligence. It is necessary to establish that the adverse outcome would not have occurred as a result of the natural progression of the disease, and was not a foreseeable and accepted complication of treatment, despite all appropriate care. When investigating a case one will often find examples of suboptimal practice that do not impact upon outcome but investigation is still important to undertake a root cause analysis for the purpose of organizational learning.

Where injuries are caused by a failure to act, it is necessary to evaluate the likely natural progress of the untreated condition and to establish what, as a fact, would have occurred but for the negligent act. If the adverse outcome was determined before the negligent intervention, or if the adverse outcome was to have been more likely than not in any event; then the claim will fail. However, if there was a greater than 50% chance, on the balance of probability, of a good outcome but for the negligent failure to act, the patient would be successful in obtaining damages.

## 🔑 Key learning points

### Specific to the case

- The risk of stroke following TIA is in large part related to carotid stenosis, hypertension and atrial fibrillation.
- Evidence-based algorithms to can be useful in determining the appropriate urgency and venue for ongoing investigation and treatment.

### General points

- Clinical care is only negligent if a duty of care is established, that duty of care is breached, and a

foreseeable injury occurs as a result of that breach.
• The *Bolam* test assesses whether an opinion or course of action taken is supported by a responsible body of medical practitioners.

## Reference

Johnston SC, Rothwell PM, Nguyen-Huynh MN *et al.* (2007) Validation and refinement of scores to predict very early stroke risk after transient ischaemic attack. *Lancet*, 369: 283–92.

# Case 6  An opportunity missed

Samantha Jenkins, 36, has been referred to the medical take by her GP with generalized fatigue, weakness and some lumbar pain. She last felt well four or five days ago. The GP's working diagnosis is of pyelonephritis although Ms Jenkins is apyrexial and urinalysis is normal.

Dr Wilkins, the on-call registrar, takes a history from Ms Jenkins who works as a police officer and usually enjoys good health. She has a three-year-old daughter who is looked after by her mother-in-law when she is at work. Ms Jenkins has mild asthma which seems to be seasonal and she has not needed salbutamol at all in the last six months although has felt more short of breath over recent days. Ms Jenkins describes a deep aching sensation over her lumbar spine which has been present for 48 hours, and generalized weakness and lethargy. It has become a real effort to climb up and down the stairs at home, so much so that she has started to use the downstairs toilet even though her husband is in the middle of decorating the room.

Systems enquiry reveals a bout of diarrhoea ten days earlier which Ms Jenkins had put down to a take-away meal.

## What is your differential diagnosis and how will you proceed?

Dr Wilkins examines Ms Jenkins. Her nursing observations are within normal limits apart from a respiratory rate of 24 per minute. Chest, cardiovascular and abdominal examination is unremarkable. Ms Jenkins is able to stand and walk unaided. The registrar makes a diagnosis of a nonspecific viral illness and sends routine blood tests. These demonstrate a sodium level of 128 mmol but are otherwise normal. Ms Jenkins is discharged home to rest with free oral fluids and regular paracetamol.

## What are your thoughts?

Ms Jenkins represents to the Emergency Department 36 hours later, and is clerked in by Dr Al-Hamdi, a core medical trainee. Ms Jenkins states that she has become so weak that she can no longer get up from a chair. Her speech has become slurred over the last few hours. On examination, she has a respiratory rate of 30, a mild facial droop and is drooling saliva. Her chest is clear and she is generally weak although this seems most profound in the distal lower limbs. Dr Al-Hamdi is unable to elicit any deep tendon reflexes.

Dr Al-Hamdi considers the possibility of Guillain-Barré Syndrome and measures Ms Jenkins's vital capacity with a handheld spirometer. It is 0.8 L. Dr Al-Hamdi seeks an intensive care opinion and Ms Jenkins is transferred to the intensive care unit for observation. Whilst there, a lumbar puncture is performed and intravenous immunoglobulin administered. Three hours after admission, Ms Jenkins is intubated because of a deterioration in vital capacity.

Ms Jenkins spends two weeks in the intensive care unit and requires a tracheostomy. She subsequently spends three months in neurological rehabilitation before discharge home. A year later, she continues to make progress, but to date she has only been able to undertake office-based duties for the police.

## Expert opinion

Although the diagnosis of Guillain-Barré syndrome was eventually made and Ms Jenkins survived, it is possible that she may have followed a more benign course had her illness been recognized earlier and appropriate treatment (IVIG / plasma exchange) been instituted earlier. She might have avoided an ITU admission and her functional status at one year may have been better.

When a differential diagnosis is made always focus on those elements of the history or examination and investigations which don't 'fit'. So, why was a previously well 36-year-old woman with an adequate blood pressure tachypnoeic, hyponatraemic, and subsequently unable to walk? One wonders by what mechanism Dr Wilkins

*Avoiding Errors in Adult Medicine*, First Edition. Ian P. Reckless, D. John M. Reynolds, Sally Newman, Joseph E. Raine, Kate Williams and Jonathan Bonser.
© 2013 John Wiley & Sons, Ltd. Published 2013 by John Wiley & Sons, Ltd.

thought a nonspecific viral illness was causing these problems.

Guillain-Barré syndrome can present in a very nonspecific manner and it is sufficiently unusual that most receiving doctors in ED or emergency assessment units may not have it foremost in their minds. The average-sized hospital in the UK will deal with only around five cases a year.

Back pain is a feature of Guillain-Barré syndrome and reflects the presence of nerve root inflammation. The typical history is of ascending distal weakness with paraesthesiae and autonomic features are common. CSF examination usually reveals an elevated protein without a significant white cell count.

When Ms Jenkins was first seen, the assessment was incomplete and her classical symptoms (even though nonspecific) were not recognized for what they were. The clinical features may progress rapidly and lead to respiratory failure as respiratory muscles become affected.

Delayed treatment for Guillain-Barré syndrome is associated with a poor outcome. Ms Jenkins may have a case to seek financial recompense for any lost earnings.

## ⚠️ Legal comment

Reimbursement of past and future loss of earnings would be included in the schedule of loss compiled by Ms Jenkins's solicitors in any legal claim. If liability is admitted at an early stage of investigation by the NHS Litigation Authority on behalf of the Trust, an interim award of damages for immediate past loss of earnings may be made to ease the financial hardship in which Ms Jenkins and her family find themselves. Ms Jenkins will of course be entitled to statutory sick pay during the initial time she is in hospital, but full pay can continue for public sector workers up to a period of six months. It is now a year since the initial incident and she has not yet returned to active police duties.

The intention of compensation is to place the claimant, so far as money is able, back in the position she would have been in, but for the negligent act. Her significant compensation is divided into general damages and special damages. Her general damages are for her pain, suffering and loss of amenity attributable to the injury. Calculation is based on annual Judicial Studies Board Guidelines, which set out a range of settlements for different types of injuries, from within which awards for a particular injury are selected. In addition, case law is used to establish or refute a particular point within any guideline range.

Special damages are losses specific to the claimant which are directly attributable to the negligence. Past losses, such as loss of earnings, can be calculated accurately whereas future losses are hypothetical. Interest on past losses are recoverable from the date of injury to the date of settlement or trial. Significant injury will potentially impact upon a patient throughout her lifetime. Although the total amount of losses calculated at the time of settlement of the claim, the patient has immediate benefit of the compensation which, but for the injury, would have taken a life term to earn.

Although Ms Jenkins may have recovered from the immediate effects of her injury by the date of settlement she may still be at a disadvantage (i.e. she has not returned to full police duties and there is a partial continuing loss of earnings, for example, through loss of overtime work). She may well be disadvantaged if in the future she were to lose her current job and find herself on the open labour market. Damages may be recovered for the weakening of Ms Jenkins's competitive position in the labour market, it does not matter that there is no immediate loss.

Ms Jenkins is also entitled to be compensated for her loss of capacity to undertake housework and to care for her child during the time when she was critically ill and for the fact that her mother-in-law looked after Ms Jenkins's three-year-old daughter more than usual. During this same time period Ms Jenkins will not have been in a position to undertake the usual contribution to the family's home life (for example, cooking and cleaning). These losses can be claimed by reference to what equivalent commercial costs would have been for a cleaner with a discount to acknowledge that these services were provided by Ms Jenkins to her close family. If Ms Jenkins' husband, as a nonprofessional, has provided care, this can also be compensated under the principles established by the case of *Housecroft v Burnett* where the needs of an injured patient have been supplied by a relative without regard to monetary reward. In this case, the loss is calculated by either the market value to employ professional help or if Mr Jenkins has given up work to look after his wife, he would have incurred actual loss of earnings.

## ⚠️ Key learning points

### General points
- Financial compensation is calculated with regard to both actual and hypothetical earnings.

# Case 7 Better late than never

Jimmy Irvine, a 38-year-old man with learning difficulties, hypothyroidism and congenital heart disease is brought to the Emergency Department by his father with a 48 hour history of lethargy, fever, myalgia, headache and anorexia. He is usually cheerful and interactive and has a passion for his local football team, attending all home matches and running the line for the U16 team. The casualty officer who sees him notes that he is sweaty, tachypnoeic and un-cooperative with examination. His oxygen saturations are 89% on room air but Mr Irvine is known to have a right to left shunt and has previously been noted to be hypoxic when well.

## What is your differential diagnosis?

The casualty officer believes that Mr Irvine has a lower respiratory tract infection. However, his chest X-ray is clear and the diagnosis is revised to that of a viral illness. The casualty officer advises oral fluids and paracetamol and discharges Mr Irvine to his father's care.

Three days later, Mr Irvine is brought back to the Emergency Department. His symptoms have continued but now he has now developed urinary incontinence and has been complaining of nausea. Mr Irvine is intermittently drowsy and aggressive. His temperature is 37.7°C and his pulse is 106 per minute. Blood pressure is maintained and saturations are 82% on air, rising to 86% with a non-rebreathe mask.

## What investigations would you pursue and what management steps would you institute?

The medical registrar prescribes ceftriaxone and contacts colleagues in ICU in order to arrange for Mr Irvine to be intubated prior to a brain CT scan and lumbar puncture. The anaesthetist is initially reluctant to intubate Mr Irvine on account of his central cyanosis and the fact that a decision had apparently been made several years prior that Mr Irvine was not to undergo cardiac

surgery. Mr Irvine then has a brief seizure and is intubated to secure his airway.

The CT scan demonstrates significant obstructive hydrocephalus with meningeal enhancement and an external ventricular drain is inserted by the neurosurgeon on-call. CSF analysis demonstrates the presence of over a thousand polymorphs. CSF protein is elevated. No organisms are seen. Subsequently *Streptococcus constellatus* is grown from the CSF.

Mr Irvine has a stormy course, requiring several external ventricular drains followed by a VP shunt and a subsequent revision. A TOE confirms a significant right to left shunt. Mr Irvine is in hospital for over three months but ultimately returns home. His function is never quite as before and Mr Irvine's elderly parents find the burden of caring for him increasingly difficult to manage. They enlist the support of a private carer on weekday afternoons to provide them with some respite.

Eight months later, the hospital receives a letter from an independent advocate asking the Trust to explain the delay in diagnosis and to state whether, if the diagnosis had been made earlier, the outcome may have been better.

## How do you think the trust should reply?

Clinicians in the Trust argue that the natural history of *Streptococcus constellatus* meningo-encephalitis is very difficult to define, particularly in a patient with learning difficulties prior to the event. They consider that Mr Irvine has had a very good outcome given his original presentation.

Trust managers commission an independent external review of the case. The reviewer's opinion was that (1) initial assessment of Mr Irvine in the Emergency Department was suboptimal and did not take adequate account of his communication difficulties, and (2) had Mr Irvine been given appropriate antibiotics on the day of presentation, the outcome would likely have been better, obstructive hydrocephalus may not

*Avoiding Errors in Adult Medicine*, First Edition. Ian P. Reckless, D. John M. Reynolds, Sally Newman, Joseph E. Raine, Kate Williams and Jonathan Bonser.
© 2013 John Wiley & Sons, Ltd. Published 2013 by John Wiley & Sons, Ltd.

have developed and the he may not have required any neurosurgical intervention with the long-term morbidity that this can carry.

The NHS Litigation Authority negotiates an out-of-court settlement on behalf of the Trust.

## 🔎 Expert opinion

The diagnosis in this case was undoubtedly delayed. Although it can be difficult to obtain a comprehensive conventional history from patients with communication difficulties of any sort, Mr Irvine was clearly septic at presentation. The casualty officer was keen to attribute the source of infection to the chest on the basis of hypoxia. Even when this was not supported by the evidence (he was known to have hypoxemia when well, and no evidence of focal consolidation on the chest radiograph), the casualty officer did not attempt to go back to the beginning.

When communication is difficult and the clinical picture is complicated by pre-existing disease (in this case congenital heart disease) it can be very difficult to reach a satisfactory diagnosis immediately and a period of observation may bring some clarity. If the diagnosis is not clear at the outset then say so – putting a firm label on a problem which is in reality unclear is unhelpful and can close minds to other more likely possibilities.

Although ultimately events dictated that Mr Irvine required intubation as an emergency, initial discussions around his appropriateness for level 3 (ICU) care seem to have been rather confrontational. It was readily evident that Mr Irvine's usual quality of life was good and that the current illness was acute and potentially reversible.

As alluded to by the independent expert asked by the Trust to review the case, it is only possible to conclude that Mr Irvine's outcome may well have been better had the diagnosis been made earlier.

## ⚖️ Legal comment

Although initial contact may have been made by an ICAS advocate, the complexity of causation and the need for expert evidence in assessing the future care requirements, means that settlement would not be by way of the complaints process but by a clinical negligence claim. Expert evidence would be required on the issue of causation to assess Mr Irvine's previous capabilities compared to his current and likely future mental capacity caused by the seizure and hydrocephalus.

The purpose of the formal NHS complaints process is to provide a factual explanation of what has happened. The complaints process cannot make an assessment of liability and complex assessment of past and future financial losses. The complaints process can provide reimbursement of minor out-of-pocket expenses. Although small ex-gratia payments (i.e. those made without an admission of liability can be made under the NHS complaints process), in a complex causal case the significant damages assessment is best undertaken in accordance with the quantum principles of a civil negligence claim.

The Trust would no doubt use the independent external review to assist in replying to Mr Irvine's family's concerns under the NHS complaints process. The complaint letter of response should provide an open and honest explanation for the factual chain of events but should avoid any admission of legal liability.

There is no prohibition to a parallel complaint investigation with a potential clinical negligence claim, provided the information provided to the complainant under the NHS complaints process does not adversely impact or does not adversely prejudice the Trust's ability to defend a clinical negligence claim. This should be discussed by the Trust's complaints manager and legal manager.

In accordance with the Civil Procedure Rules, an offer of settlement can be made by either party prior to trial by way of a Part 36 offer. In this case, if accepted by the solicitors acting for Mr Irvine, the settlement would be subject to a court approval order since Mr Irvine does not have capacity to control his own financial affairs. A Part 8 Hearing is the court's way of ensuring a fair settlement and to protect the interests of the vulnerable adult.

The solicitors acting for Mr Irvine will need to obtain expert evidence with regard to the impact of the delay in diagnosis on Mr Irvine's mental capacity and his care requirements. If the level of care provided by Mr Irvine's parents has increased substantially this will need to be factored into the claim for past losses and indeed the future losses itemized in the schedule of damages may well feature professional costs and the increased need for external care support for Mr Irvine for the rest of his life (see Case 6 for further explanation of the calculation of past and future losses).

## ⚠️ Key learning points

### Specific to the case
• Collateral history can be vital in reaching a diagnosis.
• Where there is a paucity of information, it is wise to adopt a more cautious management plan and

maintain an open differential diagnosis until information becomes available.

### General points
• Small ex-gratia payments can be made through the NHS complaints process.
• A modest change in functional status may have major ramifications for care costs over time.

## Further reading

Department of Health (2008) Healthcare for all: report of the independent inquiry into access to healthcare for people with learning disabilities. Chair: Sir Jonathan Michael. Crown. http://www.dh.gov.uk/en/Publicationsandstatistics/Publications/PublicationsPolicyAndGuidance/DH_099255 [last accessed 18 March 2012]

# Case 8 Man down

Mr Brown, a 46-year-old air traffic controller, awakes one morning at 4.45 am and gets ready to start his early morning shift. He usually cycles the six miles to the control centre but today it is raining heavily. Mr Brown showers and dresses before phoning a colleague, Nick, at 5.05 to ask for a lift to work.

Nick arrives at Mr Brown's house at 5.35, sends him a text and waits outside in the car. At 5.40, he becomes inpatient and knocks on the front door. There is no answer. Nick looks through the letter box and just as he is about to shout for Mr Brown, he catches a glimpse of a foot poking out beyond the bottom of the kitchen door. Mr Brown has collapsed in the kitchen. Nick immediately calls the ambulance and tries to gain entry through a ground floor window whilst waiting for them.

The ambulance technicians arrive at the house at 6.05. On assessment, they find Mr Brown to be mute. He has a dense right-sided weakness and appears inattentive to that side. Mr Brown is found to have an irregular pulse and a blood pressure of 172/90 mmHg. The ambulance takes him to the emergency department of the local hospital where he arrives at 6.40.

## What would you do now?

The triage nurse arranges for Mr Brown to be admitted to the 'majors' area for assessment. Nursing staff place him on a cardiac monitor and send routine blood to the laboratory. An ECG confirms AF. An ST2 trainee assesses Mr Brown at 7.10 am and makes a provisional diagnosis of a stroke. He requests a CT scan of the brain to take place that day and asks the bed manager to organize a bed on the stroke unit. Mr Brown is placed nil by mouth on account of impaired swallowing.

The CT subsequently confirms a left total anterior circulation infarction. Mr Brown spends a total of four months in hospital and makes a reasonable recovery. His mobility improves such that he is able to walk without

aids. However, he continues to have significant issues with expressive dysphasia and a homonymous hemianopia persists. He remains in atrial fibrillation and is commenced on warfarin.

## What do you think of Mr Brown's management?

Nine months following discharge, the Chief Executive receives a letter from a solicitor representing Mr Brown. The letter requests copies of Mr Brown's hospital notes and any stroke protocols in use at the Trust at the time of Mr Brown's original admission. The solicitor states that a negligence claim is being pursued against the Trust as thrombolytic therapy was not offered to Mr Brown when he had presented to hospital 95 minutes following the onset of stroke symptoms.

## Expert opinion

Mr Brown presented to hospital within three hours of symptom onset as evidenced by his having been able to shower, dress and converse normally on the telephone with Nick. The time of symptom onset must lie between 5.05 and 5.35 am. Thrombolytic therapy is licensed in acute ischaemic stroke if commenced within the first four and a half hours from symptom onset. Thrombolytic therapy is known to reduce long-term disability levels following stroke although mortality rates are not affected.

The National Institute for Health and Care Excellence undertook a technology appraisal of thrombolytic therapy in acute ischaemic stroke in 2007 and approved the use of thrombolysis for acute stroke. The NHS is required by Government to provide funding and resource for NICE approved technologies within three months of a recommendation.

Mr Brown's care has been substandard on account of the omission of an evidence-based intervention. A case

*Avoiding Errors in Adult Medicine*, First Edition. Ian P. Reckless, D. John M. Reynolds, Sally Newman, Joseph E. Raine, Kate Williams and Jonathan Bonser.
© 2013 John Wiley & Sons, Ltd. Published 2013 by John Wiley & Sons, Ltd.

could be brought against the local service commissioners for failing to provide the expected level of service.

## ⚠ Legal comment

Mr Brown arrived in the Emergency Department at 6.40 am and if thrombolytic therapy had been administered within the first four and a half hours, this may have limited the extent of infarction. However, the requirement to prove a causal link between the clinical outcome and negligent omission to instigate thrombolytic therapy presents a hurdle to the patient bringing an action in clinical negligence.

Even when there has been a Breach of Duty (i.e. in this case a failure to follow an NHS core standard) expert evidence will be required as to whether there would have been a greater than 50% chance of a good outcome but for the negligent failure to provide the thrombolytic therapy. What would Mr Brown's outcome have been if he had been provided with thrombolytic therapy? Would his level of disability have been similar in any event?

In this case, if a pleaded claim was brought on the basis that harm resulted from a transgression of a protocol (or a failure to follow accepted guidance), without good reason, then the claim is very likely to succeed.

NHS Acute Services are currently commissioned by the local Primary Care Trust (PCT). The role of the PCT and its implication as a potential co-defendant will depend on the facts of the case. For example has the PCT given clear instructions to the NHS Trust and the need to implement the core standard? If so, there would be limited grounds for legal challenge of the role of commissioner. It may be that the PCT has debated and consulted on how to allocate its local resources and promoted other health programmes in preference to implementing thrombolysis for stroke: if so, its decision-making processes may be open to challenge by way of judicial review as a public authority.

What happens if the core standard is not applied to your local population? What happens if there are two competing core standards for resources? Is there a documented audit trail of the local decision-making process for exceptions to implementation of core standards for the Trust patient population?

The Health Act 1989 imposes a statutory duty on PCTs and NHS Trusts to monitor and improve the quality of healthcare. The claim against the NHS Trust will relate to the actions of its employees under the principle of vicarious liability. The case against the PCT for failing to provide the expected levels of service will seek to look at the reasons why. Was it because of insufficient funding or insufficient monitoring? If the core standard has not been implemented for reasons of funding or alleged maladministration, the appropriate legal process would not be an action in tort. Instead, a patient should seek judicial review of the rationality of the decision-making of the PCT. However, claims based upon failure to provide a service and insufficient funding are less likely to succeed and in general the courts are reluctant to interfere with decisions taken in good faith on the allocations of scarce resources by local commissioners.

The aim of compensation is described in some detail in Case 6. Compensation is likely to be structured by way of periodical payments since this ensures a more accurate annual assessment of care needs. It also often makes for better value for money and ensures that all funds remain within the NHS until the next annual periodical payment; as opposed to paying a lump sum upfront to Mr Brown which takes this money out of NHS circulation. Expert evidence will also be required about Mr Brown's normal life expectancy prior to the incident compared with his life expectancy after the stroke.

---

## 🔑 Key learning points

### Specific to the case

• Thrombolysis is an evidence-based treatment in acute ischaemic stroke which can reduce disability without impact on mortality rates.
• NHS organizations have a duty to provide treatments that have been approved through the NICE Technology Appraisal process.

### General points

• Whilst NHS standards set important expectations for care in the NHS, to date the courts have been reluctant to become involved in relation to resource allocation decisions.

# Case 9  Cry wolf

James O'Connell is a 31 year old man with a long history of cigarette, marijuana, alcohol and opioid drug abuse, who in the last 12 months has attended the emergency department on at least 30 occasions saying he has taken an overdose or that he has severe chest pain and needs to be admitted to hospital. He is known to be infected with hepatitis C and he has an abnormal chest X-ray with pleural thickening at the left base, possibly following chest trauma. His ECG has high ST take off in the anterior leads but is otherwise normal and there is a copy on file in the departmental folder for comparison when he comes in complaining of chest pain.

He is often intoxicated when he arrives late at night but he is never abusive to staff who know him well and he almost always takes his own discharge the next morning after breakfast. Numerous attempts have been made to change his behaviour and the psychiatry liaison team have labelled him as having a personality disorder. In recent weeks his attendances have become less frequent and he seems to be more content since he has been sleeping at the local night shelter.

On Friday night he arrives in the emergency department and tells the nursing sister on duty that he has chest pain and feels very sick and dizzy.

## What course of action would be appropriate for the triage nurse?

The sister knows him of old and tells the emergency department registrar that 'Jimmy's back', writing in the notes 'multiple attender, complaining of chest pain again'. She records the BP at 96/65, heart rate 98, respiratory rate 26, oxygen saturations 91% on air, but she does not register that these are abnormal or that they should trigger prompt investigation.

The registrar, Dr Proudfoot, has met Mr O'Connell previously and after some friendly banter he undertakes a cursory examination. He notes there is dullness at the base of the left lung but when he reviews the old chest X-rays he assumes this is longstanding. Dr Proudfoot tells Mr O'Connell that this time the hospital is very busy and he cannot just come in for a bed for the night. He tells him to go back to the night shelter and moves on to his next patient without writing adequate notes or addressing the obvious physiological abnormalities. Dr Proudfoot simply writes 'ISQ – not for admission' in the notes before moving on to the next patient in the queue.

## What do you think about Dr Proudfoot's actions?

Jimmy hangs around the waiting area and continues to complain that he feels dizzy and unwell but no more observations are performed and he is encouraged to leave by the security staff. He returns to the night shelter and next morning he does not get up and staff check on him and find him to be very pale, sweaty and monosyllabic. They wonder if he is withdrawing from alcohol but an experienced volunteer care worker is concerned and arranges an ambulance to take Mr O'Connell back to hospital. When he arrives he is clearly very sick with a blood pressure of 60 mmHg systolic, a heart rate of 140 and unrecordable oxygen saturations. He is given intravenous fluids and antibiotics and is taken to the intensive care unit for inotropic support. Despite intensive support he succumbs to overwhelming staphylococcal infection associated with an infected groin wound where he had been injecting his heroin.

His case is referred to the coroner who is concerned that inadequate care was provided and staff dismissed Mr O'Connell's complaints because he had 'cried wolf' so often.

## Expert opinion

Every Acute Medical Unit and Emergency Department will have its cohort of regulars who are very well known to the staff. Some have serious problems which result in

*Avoiding Errors in Adult Medicine*, First Edition. Ian P. Reckless, D. John M. Reynolds, Sally Newman, Joseph E. Raine, Kate Williams and Jonathan Bonser.
© 2013 John Wiley & Sons, Ltd. Published 2013 by John Wiley & Sons, Ltd.

frequent exacerbations (e.g. brittle diabetics, asthmatics and patients with COPD and angina) and knowing them well allows prompt action to be taken and early recognition of when they are even more sick than usual. Other frequent attenders have anxiety or personality problems and they are at particular risk of not being taken seriously.

Few doctors respond well to being deliberately misled by people who have different motivations for seeking admission than the average patient, and it is all too easy to allow personal feelings to override a dispassionate professional assessment. That is not to say that every such patient who complains recurrently of chest pain and breathlessness (caused by hyperventilation) should get chest X-rays, and a CTPA – but as in Mr O'Connell's case you should never ignore clear warning signs that there may be a more serious problem on this occasion.

Always ask yourself 'how do I explain the low oxygen saturation or the persistent tachycardia?' and if you cannot logically do so then do not ignore it. It should be no skin off your nose if the next morning when the old notes arrive that you find you have done what the last ten junior doctors did and you admitted someone unnecessarily. You have to take people at face value, particularly when you are inexperienced. The competence and confidence to discharge this group of patients promptly comes with experience – make sure you develop the competence before the confidence. At all times maintain appropriate professional behaviour, examine and assess patients thoroughly, irrespective of their background or past behaviour. A history of previous problematic behaviour does not confer immunity to subsequent serious illness.

## ⚖ Legal comment

In accordance with the Human Rights Act 1998 and NHS policies supporting equality and diversity, a frequent attender is owed the same duty of care as any other patient to have a full clinical assessment of the reasons behind his attendance at the Emergency Department on each occasion that he presents. Such a cursory examination is a breach of duty of care and was compounded by lack of documentation. The decision to discharge was premature and not based on a full clinical assessment of the presenting clinical complaint. The previous or recent past medical history would not provide any adequate defence to a civil litigation claim.

The coroner will be looking at the chronological chain of factual events leading to the patient's death and as such, the factual evidence of staff under oath, would demonstrate that they had not undertaken a full and proper assessment. To avoid a Rule 43 Letter, or adverse criticism from the coroner, the Trust would need to evidence organizational learning by way of patient pathway protocols which staff should follow with regard to making a diagnosis and seeking a more senior opinion if required.

There are cases when frequent attenders are present on Trust premises with no presenting clinical condition. Any verbal or physical harassment should be documented in accordance with the Trust's Zero Tolerance Policy since such documentation in the patient's healthcare records and Incident Report Forms will provide background evidence for the Trust should it wish to take forward prosecution under the Harassment Act 1997, whereby three previous examples of pre-existing behaviour are required. An injunction can be considered if a patient persistently attends Trust premises without a genuine presenting clinical condition but any Injunction Order will make it clear that the patient is still entitled to attend Trust premises for clinically diagnosed emergency treatment. Information sharing with other public health bodies and local authorities may demonstrate that the frequent attender's behaviour is also having impact on other public authority resources. In these cases joint application to court for an injunction may assist.

## ⚖ Key learning points

### General points
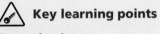
- Have regard to your position on the spectrum from cavalier under-investigation through to defensive medicine.

# Case 10 Not a leg to stand on

Rashid Khan is a 73-year-old man with angina, type 2 diabetes and diabetic nephropathy who has been living alone since the death of his wife two years ago. His daughter has become concerned that he is becoming less mobile and is having difficulty looking after himself. She calls in to see him and finds him to be mildly confused. She also notes that he has been incontinent of urine. The GP is asked to visit and he finds Mr Khan to have a temperature of 38.5 °C and he refers him to the acute medical take with a presumptive diagnosis of urinary infection.

It has been a very busy intake and Dr Jones, a medical consultant is triaging patients in a cubicle on the AMU. She takes a history from Mr Khan who denies much is wrong, but Dr Jones notes the continuing pyrexia and finds coarse crepitations at the right lung base. She asks for a chest X-ray and a urine dip, some electrolytes and blood cultures. Mr Khan's right leg is bandaged and Dr Jones asks what the problem with the foot is and is told that there is an ulcer at the ankle which the district nurse has been dressing. Dr Jones does not take the dressing down but makes a note to do so later on the post take ward round.

## Is this a reasonable course of action?

Two hours later Dr Jones reviews Mr Khan and looks at the chest X-ray which she feels shows some patchy changes at the right base and she commences oral co-amoxiclav. The blood tests she did show a creatinine of 190 mmol/l, the CRP is greater than 160 and the blood glucose is 13.7 mmol/l. The urine dip shows ++ protein but no leucocytes or nitrites. A diagnosis of pneumonia is made and Dr Jones asks the nursing staff to keep a close eye on the blood glucose and to take the dressings down that evening. Before this can be done a bed becomes available on one of the medical wards and Mr Khan is transferred.

At midday the next day the medical registrar, Dr Pandher looks in on Mr Khan who seems cheerful and his temperature is now 37.5 °C. The blood glucose remains around 14 mmol/l and no further action is taken. Dr Pandher leaves a note for the weekend cover team to ask them to review Mr Khan and ensure his diabetic control is adequate.

On Monday, Dr Jones and her team see Mr Khan again and Dr Jones is concerned that Mr Khan appears to have deteriorated. His temperature is still 38.0 °C and he is now unable to mobilize because he is weak and his right foot is mildly painful. Dr Jones takes the dressings on the foot down and is alarmed to find a very deep, foul smelling and necrotic wound on the heel which appears to involve the bone. She realizes that the dressing is the same one Mr Khan had when he was admitted four days earlier. An urgent MRI of the foot is arranged and the plastic surgery team are asked to come to advise. The scan confirms a diagnosis of osteomyelitis and a shard of glass is found in the wound. Despite two attempts at debridement and the use of broad spectrum antibiotics, it is not possible to salvage Mr Khan's leg and 10 days after admission he undergoes a below knee amputation and after a further prolonged attempt at rehabilitation arrangements are made for him to sell his home and move to a nursing home.

## Was this preventable?

Mr Khan's daughter asks why the infection was not detected earlier and Dr Jones explains that she asked for the dressings to be taken down on the day of admission but a combination of pressure of work and the fact that Mr Khan was moved to the ward meant that the message did not get passed on. Dr Jones apologizes and acknowledges she should have done this herself in view of the clear history of diabetes with microvascular complications. On review of her notes they are found to be brief and do not show any record that she looked for signs of peripheral neuropathy or peripheral vascular disease. She felt she had made a diagnosis of pneumonia and did not look for further problems.

*Avoiding Errors in Adult Medicine*, First Edition. Ian P. Reckless, D. John M. Reynolds, Sally Newman, Joseph E. Raine, Kate Williams and Jonathan Bonser.
© 2013 John Wiley & Sons, Ltd. Published 2013 by John Wiley & Sons, Ltd.

The family decide to seek compensation on the grounds that the delay in diagnosis affected the outcome and made amputation inevitable. If the infection had been picked up earlier he might have been spared the operation and could have been able to return home instead of having to pay for a nursing home.

## ⚗ Expert opinion

Most doctors practising acute medicine will readily relate to Dr Jones' situation. She was doing the best of a bad job during a busy on-call and making brief triage assessments of the patients presenting to the medial take. Her assessments were not as thorough as they might have been but her purpose was triage not to undertake definitive clerking. Each stage of the delay to inspecting Mr Khan's foot can easily be explained away but when taken together the result was catastrophic. Dr Jones' error was inadequate handover – it is perfectly acceptable not to have taken down the dressings in the first hour or so of admission but failure to appreciate the potential severity of diabetic foot infection is a recurring theme in medico-legal cases.

Always examine what lies beneath dressings and difficult to remove clothing, especially where there is a high index of suspicion of infection.

## ⚖ Legal comment

Breach of duty will be difficult to defend in this civil clinical negligence claim. Dr Jones did not remove the dressing at the time of initial assessment. The request for nursing staff to take the dressing down appears to have been a verbal instruction as opposed to one documented in the healthcare records. Further time is lost over the weekend and the failure in the interim by the nursing team to review the dressing represents care which falls below acceptable standards. Mr Khan has been left with a foreign body in his foot whilst under the care of the medical team. The issue of causation will be the key ground for dispute in the civil claim. To what extent would the below knee amputation have been avoided if the dressings had been removed on the evening of admission and immediate treatment undertaken to remove the shard of glass, to debride and to prescribe broad spectrum antibiotics?

Expert evidence will be required as to whether the delay in assessment by the medical team has affected the outcome. This will be a high value claim with significant compensation given the impact on Mr Khan's mobility, and the difference between prognosis had the below knee amputation been avoided. Future care is usually the most expensive part of a future damages claim. Providing nursing care and adaption of an existing home would not be as costly as nursing home fees and the impact of having to sell Mr Khan's house. This case highlights the importance of clear documentation of communication of requests for actions to be taken between different parts of the healthcare multi-disciplinary team and to provide later evidence of clinical decision making, escalation and expectations. The defendant in the claim will be the NHS Trust on behalf of all its employees.

Review by the Trust's clinical risk team for root causes should also include training/reflection by the medical and nursing staff involved on the failure to provide adequate care. Dr Jones' actions are further impaired by a lack of documentation regarding her clinical examination and consideration of differential diagnoses. Depending on the expert evidence in regard to causation there may be grounds for obtaining a causation discount. If the expert advice is that even if the wound had been examined at initial admission and appropriate treatment instigated, there would have been no difference in outcome, this can be used as a basis, following meeting of experts, to negotiate a discounted settlement.

## ⚗ Key learning points

### General points

• All patients should receive a thorough assessment appropriate to their presenting problem on arrival in hospital.

• Patients with diabetes who have existing problems with skin damage in the feet are at very high risk of serious complications. Always ensure dressings are taken down as soon as possible, no matter how inconvenient it is.

# Section 2: Unexpected death: the coronial system and clinical risk management

# Case 11  A doubly bad outcome

Mrs Benjamin is a 34-year-old woman who has been referred to the medical assessment unit by her GP with a 48-hour history of breathlessness. She is short of breath on minimal exertion but there are no other associated symptoms – specifically no cough or chest pain. Mrs Benjamin is an occasional smoker and has no personal history of respiratory disease. She returned from honeymoon in the Maldives six weeks ago where she had developed a swollen left calf shortly after stepping on some coral. This had improved over a week or so. She is seen in the assessment unit by Dr Talbot, the on-call SHO. Mrs Benjamin seems anxious and remarks to Dr Talbot that her grandfather died in an adjacent bay two years ago.

## What is the differential diagnosis and how would you investigate her complaint?

Mrs Benjamin's respiratory rate at rest is 26 min$^{-1}$ and oxygen saturations on air are 98%. The chest is clear with breath sounds heard throughout. Dr Talbot feels that it is important to rule out a pulmonary embolus. She sends off a panel of blood tests including a D-dimer and requests a chest radiograph before assessing another acutely unwell patient whilst awaiting results. Half an hour later, Dr Talbot is called by the radiographer who informs her that Mrs Benjamin is tearful and refusing to have a chest radiograph as she is 14/40 pregnant.

## How does this new information influence your management plan?

Mrs Benjamin tells Dr Talbot that she became pregnant on her second cycle of IVF and is terrified of the potential effect of radiation on the pregnancy. Dr Talbot explains that a chest radiograph involves a very modest exposure and the effects of this can be further mitigated by abdominal shielding. Simultaneously, Mrs

Benjamin's blood results are available showing a normal CRP and D-dimer. Dr Talbot and Mrs Benjamin agree that she will have a chest radiograph to rule out the possibility of a pneumothorax but that further ionizing radiation (for example, CTPA) will not be necessary in view of the D-dimer result. Mrs Benjamin's radiograph is entirely normal and she is discharged home with Dr Talbot's reassurance.

## What are your thoughts upon Dr Talbot's management plan?

Six days later, Mrs Benjamin collapses at home. An ambulance is called and she is found to be in cardiac arrest. Resuscitation efforts continue en-route to the emergency department. Twenty minutes after arrival there, in the absence of a return of spontaneous circulation, the resuscitation attempt is called off.

A coroner's inquest is held and although Mrs Benjamin is found to have died from natural causes (pulmonary embolism), the coroner criticizes the Trust for a failure to appropriately investigate Mrs Benjamin during her attendance to the AMU.

## Expert opinion

Mrs Benjamin presented with acute shortness of breath with clear tachypnoea and no associated symptoms to suggest an infective aetiology. Even without the history of pregnancy, the presentation along with the history of a long haul flight and leg symptoms made it imperative to rule out venous thrombo-embolism (VTE). A D-dimer was not appropriate given the high probability of thromboembolic disease. The subsequent disclosure of pregnancy and IVF treatment heightens the chances of VTE still further.

Dr Talbot did not achieve the appropriate balance between risks and benefits. Fatal VTE is more common during pregnancy and puerperium than in age matched

*Avoiding Errors in Adult Medicine*, First Edition. Ian P. Reckless, D. John M. Reynolds, Sally Newman, Joseph E. Raine, Kate Williams and Jonathan Bonser.
© 2013 John Wiley & Sons, Ltd. Published 2013 by John Wiley & Sons, Ltd.

controls. The consequences of missed or poorly managed VTE are also greater with two lives at risk. Based on the history, Mrs Benjamin should have been counselled that the benefits of a definitive test to confirm or rule out VTE outweighed the risks. Non-ionizing tests including lower limb Doppler and echocardiography could have formed part of the investigative strategy although had they been normal, Mrs Benjamin should have been advised to continue to perfusion scanning or CTPA according to local protocols.

Dr Talbot failed to use the D-dimer test in an evidence-based manner. She failed to enquire as to whether her patient was pregnant prior to requesting the use of ionizing radiation. Dr Talbot also failed to seek expert advice from senior physicians, radiologists or obstetricians. This points to a lack of awareness of her own limitations and competencies, or a systematic problem in the hospital if junior doctors are left to 'fend for themselves'.

The confidential enquiries into maternal death (CEMD) have long reported avoidable death through VTE. Many of the features of this case – including a well-meaning desire to minimize risk for mother and unborn child – are common to those cases reported in CEMD.

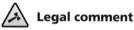 **Legal comment**

Proceedings in the coroner's court are governed by the Coroner's Act 1988 supplemented by the Coroner's Rules 1984 (as amended). The duty of the coroner is restricted to investigations of certain deaths. He is charged with the duty to make inquiry where there is reasonable cause to suspect that a person's death was either violent or unnatural, sudden and of unknown cause. Whilst doctors commonly sign a death certificate this document certifies the cause of death only. The registrar of births and deaths issues the actual legal death certificate. There is no obligation on doctors to report deaths to the coroner but it is sensible to do so. A death should be reported to a coroner in the following circumstances:

- The cause of death is unknown.
- The doctor has not attended the patient during his last illness.
- The doctor neither attended the patient during the last 14 days before death nor saw the patient's body after death.
- Death occurred during an operation or before recovery from the effects of an anaesthetic.

- Death was caused by industrial disease or poisoning.
- Death was believed to be unnatural or caused by violence, neglect or abortion.

Informal consultation with the coroner is vital to clarify whether or not a patient death should be reported.

The coroner has jurisdiction over a patient's body once death has been reported. He can order a post-mortem to be undertaken by a practitioner of his choice. When death occurs in the course of medical treatment, particularly if concerns have been expressed about the standard of care, an independent pathologist usually carries out the post-mortem at another location.

The inquest hearing is not a trial and the coroner's terms of reference are restricted since the coroner only considers questions about who the deceased was, and when, where, and how the deceased came to his/her death.

Where a patient's death has also resulted in a Serious Incident Requiring Investigation (SIRI) by the NHS Trust it is good practice to share the report and completed action plan with the coroner as evidence of organizational learning. Rule 43 of the Coroner's Rules 1984 enables a coroner to refer matters to the appropriate authority, if by so doing it may enable changes to be made to prevent repetition of similar fatalities. In the context of the NHS, the coroner would send a Rule 43 letter to the Chief Executive of the NHS Trust and under Rule 43A the Trust is required to provide a written response within 56 days. Any Rule 43 letters issued are automatically copied to the Ministry of Justice and appear in the Ministry of Justice's Annual Summary Report. The Care Quality Commission also monitors Rule 43 letters with regard to healthcare. The first Ministry of Justice Summary Report was published in September 2011. The report seeks to identify any emerging national trends relating to patient safety.

Against whom would a case be brought – the individual doctor or the NHS Trust? Actions in negligence require there to be a person or persons, who owe a duty of care. Where the patient has received acute NHS care, the NHS Trust is cited as the defendant. Actions against GPs will name the individual doctor as defendant. Similarly, private practitioners are pursued individually or are identified as a co-defendant with the private hospital. Where a doctor is employed by an NHS Trust then the named defendant will be the NHS Trust under the legal principle of vicarious liability.

## ⚠️ Key learning points

### Specific to the case

• When providing medical treatment to pregnant women, urgent radiological investigation should not normally be deferred. When unsure, the advice of an expert should always be sought.

• Always work closely with obstetricians when assessing pregnant patients. Even when your advice and treatment plan are appropriate, an expert in pregnancy may be able to provide a greater degree of confidence. Never underestimate in pregnancy how worrying it is to have to contemplate drug therapy and ionizing radiation.

### General points

• When they relate to NHS care, actions in negligence are typically brought against the NHS Trust and not an individual employee.

• The coroner can issue a Rule 43 letter which requires a response from the NHS Trust and will be noted by the Ministry of Justice and the Care Quality Commission.

## Further reading

Centre for Maternal and Child Enquiries (CMACE) (2011) Saving Mothers' Lives: reviewing maternal deaths to make motherhood safer: 2006–08. The Eighth Report on Confidential Enquiries into Maternal Deaths in the United Kingdom. *BJOG* 118 (Suppl. 1): 1–203.

# Case 12 Difficulty with diarrhoea

Mrs Brooks is an 84-year-old woman who is referred by her GP to the general medical take with weakness, nausea, malaise, and shortness of breath (SOB). She has been unable to cope at home because of the weakness and multiple co-morbidities which include rheumatoid arthritis, chronic renal impairment, gastro-oesophageal reflux, chronic heart failure and recurrent urinary sepsis. The current problems started three weeks earlier with urinary frequency and pyrexia for which she received a seven-day course of oral co-amoxiclav from her GP.

Her current medication is methotrexate 10 mg once a week, omeprazole 40 mg daily, furosemide 40 mg daily, lisinopril 7.5 mg daily, as well as folinic acid, co-codamol, senna and lactulose.

Dr Papadakis, the medical CT1 who first examines Mrs Brooks, finds her to be weak and frail. She is apyrexial and hypotensive with a systolic blood pressure of 95 mm Hg. She has a heart rate of 125 in atrial fibrillation. There are widespread crackles in both lung fields. The chest X-ray shows cardiomegaly and a small left pleural effusion with patchy consolidation at the right lung base. The initial blood results show she has a normochromic normocytic anaemia with a haemoglobin of 9.6 g/dl and a white blood count of 11.9. She has renal failure with a creatinine of 221 mmol/l (previously 155) and an albumin of 29 g/l. The CRP is 39. A diagnosis of heart failure and possible chest infection is made and she is commenced on intravenous cefuroxime and given an intravenous infusion of 1L of normal saline over 6 hours. She is given a loading dose of oral digoxin with a plan to continue with 62.5 micrograms daily thereafter.

## Would you have managed the situation in the same way?

On the post take ward round 2 hours later she is somewhat improved and the consultant agrees with the management plan. She is reviewed the next day (a Friday) when she is still apyrexial, her systolic blood pressure is now 120 mmHg and her apical rate has slowed to 80. She complains of some abdominal discomfort and her dose of laxative is increased.

At handover that evening the FY1 doctor identifies Mrs Brooks as a patient who is unwell and who requires review over the weekend but as she is improving no change in her management plan is communicated to the cover team.

On the Sunday evening the nurse looking after Mrs Brooks is concerned that she is less communicative and is complaining of intermittent abdominal pain. Her temperature has risen to 38.5 °C and she is once again tachycardic. The CRP taken earlier that day has risen to 140 and the albumin has fallen further to 22. The cover FY1 comes to see Mrs Brooks and is worried by the temperature, believing she has pneumonia which is not responding to antibiotics. She adds in a macrolide antibiotic to the cephalosporin and arranges a plain abdominal film because Mrs Brooks by now has a very tender abdomen and has just had two episodes of diarrhoea.

The plain abdominal film shows some colonic dilatation but no further action is taken at this stage. The next morning Mrs Brooks is very unwell and has had persistent diarrhoea overnight. Her abdomen is distended and very tender. The nurse in charge reports that the diarrhoea is very suggestive of *Clostridium difficile* infection and a stool sample is sent which confirms C difficile toxin. The result is available the next day and oral vancomycin and intravenous steroids are started but Mrs Brooks rapidly deteriorates and dies on the Tuesday night.

At the team's Mortality and Morbidity review meeting, the notes and clinical history are reassessed and the conclusion is reached that Mrs Brooks died of overwhelming *Clostridium difficile* colitis which had not been detected soon enough to allow adequate treatment. The cause of death was noted as 1a *C difficile* colitis, automatically triggering a Serious Incident Requiring Investigation (SIRI) process.

*Avoiding Errors in Adult Medicine*, First Edition. Ian P. Reckless, D. John M. Reynolds, Sally Newman, Joseph E. Raine, Kate Williams and Jonathan Bonser.
© 2013 John Wiley & Sons, Ltd. Published 2013 by John Wiley & Sons, Ltd.

## ⚠️ Expert opinion

Mrs Brooks has multiple risk factors for healthcare acquired infection and for *C difficile* in particular. She is elderly, immunosuppressed with methotrexate and has rheumatoid arthritis, she is receiving a proton pump inhibitor and she has renal impairment and heart failure. She has recently been treated with a seven-day course of co-amoxiclav and on admission to hospital was given a broad spectrum intravenous cephalosporin and later a macrolide antibiotic as well. The use of laxatives may also have been relevant.

The evidence that she had an infective problem on admission was not convincing and her symptoms were compatible with a combination of dehydration and renal impairment in the context of heart failure, anaemia, and atrial fibrillation. The use of cefuroxime was inadvisable at the outset and should have been questioned on the post take ward round. The abdominal pain, the pyrexia, the falling albumin, and the rise in the CRP are all features compatible with the onset of colitis.

*C difficile* infection is strongly associated with antibiotic usage and in this case the prescription of cefuroxime for an unproven pneumonia was very ill advised. Indeed, a seven-day course of co-amoxiclav for an uncomplicated UTI is excessive. This was further compounded by the failure to review the prescription after 24 hours and for it to continue over the weekend. Many hospitals have introduced automatic stop or review dates for intravenous antibiotics and even the simple act of writing the proposed duration of therapy on the drug chart might have empowered the cover team to have modified the prescription. The handover was inadequate – no patient should be left receiving intravenous or broad spectrum antibiotics over a weekend without being reviewed and careful plans put in place and communicated.

If *C difficile* is suspected, appropriate treatment with either vancomycin or metronidazole should commence before waiting for the results of stool sampling. Delays in starting treatment may adversely affect outcome.

A SIRI was undertaken which concluded that death was the result of *C difficile* colitis in a lady with significant risk factors. This case was one of several which occurred over a six-month period and which triggered a major review of antibiotic stewardship within the hospital, resulting in a change in antibiotic policy and a programme of education for all medical staff. Ward pharmacists were instructed to challenge prescriptions for intravenous antibiotics over 48h duration and all prescriptions of antibiotics were required to include the indication for, and duration of, antibiotic therapy. This has since been continuously audited and reported to the hospital board. The incidence of *C difficile* infection has fallen very significantly since these changes were instituted.

The Department of Health continues to closely manage rates of *C difficile* infection in the NHS in England. A heavy focus on reducing the number of cases identified may be counterproductive with *C difficile* as the detection of C toxin does not necessarily indicate disease in a patient with loose stool (rather incidental asymptomatic carriage) and these 'targets' may lead to a more conservative approach to testing for *C difficile* in general, potentially resulting in failure to diagnose in a timely fashion.

## ⚠️ Legal comment

The patient's death should also be notified to the coroner, as death was 'unnatural' (due to hospital acquired infection) and possibly neglectful if the *C difficile* colitis had not been detected soon enough to allow adequate treatment. Some of the terms in the reporting requirements of the Coroner's Act 1988, supplemented by the Coroner's Rules 1984, are imprecise, for example, 'unnatural' in the context of an elderly patient such as Mrs Brooks. When a coroner is informed of such a death, he/she has the discretion to dispense with an Inquest, with or without a post-mortem. Informal discussion with the coroner's office will clarify whether or not a patient's death should be reported.

When clinicians discuss a case 'with the coroner'; a coroner's officer usually serves as intermediary. The police previously employed coroner's officers but they are now employees of the Local Authority. They are administrators and do not have legal responsibility. Coroner's officers are usually the first point of contact in the coroner's office for advice about whether a patient's death should be formally notified to the coroner. The coroner's officer will discuss with the coroner, if required on more complex matters, and where necessary will facilitate direct communication between the coroner and the referring doctor.

If the coroner does decide to open an inquest, the SIRI report and action plan should be shared with the coroner as evidence of organizational learning and changes that have been made to antibiotic stewardship in the Trust. This may provide sufficient assurance to coroner to avoid a Rule 43 letter of steps taken to improve patient safety. It is also good practice for the patient's family to be given a copy of the SIRI report and invited to meet with appropriate clinicians/managers to discuss their concerns.

The SIRI report and action plan is also notified to the PCT and SHA. If this case is one of several in a cluster, then it is likely that this will have triggered closer monitoring under the Trust's performance contract with the PCT of the Trust's management of *C difficile* until audit results demonstrated an improvement.

All NHS Trusts also have to self-register with the Care Quality Commission to confirm the status of their compliance with infection control standards and are open to being inspected by the CQC as to the accuracy of the data provided. All NHS Trusts now require staff to undertake mandatory training in infection control to raise awareness of the potential for healthcare acquired infection.

- *C difficile* remains a common problem and is associated with high morbidity and mortality in elderly, frail patients.
- In the case of Mrs Brooks, there was an unnecessary urgency to commence 'a definitive treatment' – watching and waiting is often an appropriate approach.

### General points

- Organizations providing NHS care must comply with defined standards (for example, around infection control and relevant training) and risk their operating license where they fail to do so.
- There was a lack of senior review over the weekend –a failing which is all too common. Patient care should be the same regardless of the time or day of the week on which they are admitted – something which the NHS recognizes but struggles to deliver.

### Key learning points

#### Specific to the case

- *C difficile* should be treated when it is considered pending confirmation

### Further reading

Health & Safety Executive (2007) Investigation into a *Clostridium difficile* outbreak at Stoke Mandeville Hospital, Buckinghamshire http://www.hse.gov.uk/press/2007/e07043.htm [last accessed 01 June 2012]

# Case 13 A flu-like illness

Shaun Jones is a 34-year-old flight lieutenant in the Royal Air Force. He is generally fit and well. He is brought to the Emergency Department by his girlfriend one evening because he is pyrexial (39.2 °C) and drowsy. There are no localizing signs in respect of the fever. Mr Jones's Glasgow Coma Score is 13/15 but there is no focal neurology. His girlfriend says that he has been complaining of a flu-like illness with prominent headache that has been progressing over the last 24 hours. He has appeared confused during the course of the afternoon. Mr Jones is seen initially by Dr Smethwick, the duty consultant.

## What diagnoses should occur to Dr Smethwick?

Dr Smethwick instantly recognizes that Mr Jones is unwell and considers the diagnosis of meningitis. In addition to the fever, Mr Jones has a tachycardia and his initial blood pressure is 94 mmHg systolic. However, there is no history of photophobia or neck stiffness, and in the absence of any rash, Dr Smethwick feels an encephalitic process is more likely. In any event, Dr Smethwick sends bloods (including for culture) and immediately institutes appropriate antibiotics for meningitis, intravenous aciclovir and aggressive fluid resuscitation. He requests a CT examination of the head and refers Mr Jones on to the medical team for further management and consideration of a lumbar puncture.

## Should any other treatments have been instigated?

Mr Jones's initial treatments are commenced whilst he awaits review by the medical team. His blood pressure remains low but the nursing staff are able to maintain a systolic over 90 mmHg with liberal use of colloid. Initial blood tests from haematology show a platelet count of 43 000. Dr Smethwick (who is now busy with a trauma call) writes an entry in Mr Jones's notes cautioning against lumbar puncture until the full blood count

has been repeated. He also checks with Mr Jones's nurse that the antibiotics have been administered.

## Is there anything else that you would do?

An hour later, whilst in the CT scanner, Mr Jones has a grand mal seizure. The seizure appears to respond to intravenous lorazepam but soon recurs. Mr Jones is given further lorazepam and a phenytoin infusion is commenced. The fits continue. He is paralysed, anaesthetized and given phenobarbital before being taken to the intensive care unit. His blood pressure falls and metaraminol is administered. The effect is short-lived. Mr Jones's blood pressure continues to fall, he suffers a cardiac arrest and resuscitation attempts are unsuccessful.

Dr Smethwick and the intensive-care team discuss the cause of Mr Jones's death, and consider viral encephalitis as the most likely aetiology. Mr Jones's death is discussed with the coroner's officer and a medical certificate of cause of death (MCCD) is issued.

Five days later, Mr Jones's case is discussed at the hospital's postgraduate medical meeting. One of the consultants present suggests the diagnosis of cerebral malaria and there is a general consensus that this is a likely diagnosis.

## What should the hospital do at this stage?

The hospital contacts the coroner's office and explains the developments in relation to Mr Jones's case. The coroner opens an Inquest and orders a post-mortem examination which delays the funeral, arranged for the next day, and causes much upset to Mr Jones's family. Cerebral malaria is confirmed at post mortem.

## ⚠ Expert opinion

Mr Jones was clearly extremely ill at presentation. The prominent issues were fever, confusion and headache.

---

*Avoiding Errors in Adult Medicine*, First Edition. Ian P. Reckless, D. John M. Reynolds, Sally Newman, Joseph E. Raine, Kate Williams and Jonathan Bonser.
© 2013 John Wiley & Sons, Ltd. Published 2013 by John Wiley & Sons, Ltd.

Whilst a travel history was not offered, Mr Jones's occupation is a clear risk marker in relation to malaria. Falciparum malaria should have been high up in Dr Smethwick's differential diagnosis. Profound thrombocytopenia should also have set alarm bells ringing. Although a rare diagnosis in the United Kingdom, malaria should have been considered in the Emergency Department.

From the time of presentation to death, Mr Jones was in the hospital for only three hours. It is likely that recognition and treatment of malaria would not have altered outcome.

Dr Smethwick and the intensivists should not have completed an MCCD given that the diagnosis of encephalitis was entirely speculative. The coroner's officer should not have sanctioned certification but does not have sufficient experience or medical knowledge to realize that the explanation put forward by the clinical team was not plausible.

The hospital should count itself lucky that the coroner did not issue a Rule 43 letter criticizing their death certification processes. From April 2013, the role of Medical Examiner will be introduced across England to standardize and quality assure the death certification process. Scrutiny by a medical examiner may have been of assistance in this case.

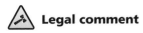 **Legal comment**

In this case, it was possible to arrange a post mortem despite the unusual circumstances. Had the patient's body been buried, the coroner may have considered the unusual step of ordering exhumation.

According to section 23 of the Coroner's Act 1998, a coroner may order by warrant the exhumation of a body if it appears that an examination of the body is necessary for the purpose of the coroner's own functions in holding an inquest or inquiring into a person's death. Such exhumations are extremely rare, with nine being ordered by coroners in England and Wales between 2006 and 2010.

Proceedings in the coroner's court are governed by The Coroner's Act 1998, supplemented by The Coroner's Rules 1984. The duty of the coroner is to investigate certain deaths when informed that the body of a person is lying in his jurisdiction and there is reasonable cause to suspect that the death:
- was violent or unnatural;
- was sudden and of unknown cause;
- occurred in prison; or
- occurred in such a place or circumstances to require a inquest.

Doctors frequently sign a 'death certificate' and this only certifies the cause of death. The legal death certificate is issued by the Registrar of Births and Deaths. There is no obligation on a doctor to report deaths to the coroner that lie within the above criteria, but it is sensible, wise and courteous to do so. The Registrar will report the death to the coroner if he is not prepared to issue a formal death certificate on the information received.

A patient's death should be reported to the coroner in the following situations:
- The cause of death is unknown.
- The doctor has not attended the patient during his last illness.
- The doctor did not attend the patient during the last 14 days of life and did not see the body after death.
- Death occurred during an operation or before recovery from the effects of the anaesthetic.
- Death was caused by an industrial disease or poisoning.
- Death is believed to be unnatural or caused by violence, neglect or abortion.

Rule 43 of the Coroner's Rules 1984 states that a coroner who believes that action should be taken to prevent the recurrence of fatalities similar to that in respect of which the inquest is being held may announce at the inquest that he is reporting the matter in writing to the 'person of authority' who may have such power to take such action. In the context of the NHS, this is the Chief Executive of the NHS Trust.

The Coroner's (Amendment) Rules 2008 introduced a new statutory duty for organizations to respond to a Rule 43 letter sent to them by a coroner. The recipient must provide a response within 56 days and this should contain details of any actions which have been or will be taken, or provide an explanation when no action is deemed necessary or appropriate.

All Rule 43 letters issued by coroners in England and Wales since 1 October 2010 have been reported to the Ministry of Justice and where the Rule 43 letter concerns a NHS public authority this has been notified to the Care Quality Commission. The first Ministry of Justice Summary Report was published in September 2011. Rule 43 letters were issued in relation to 189 inquests, relating to 86 NHS hospitals and Trusts. An analysis in relation to hospital deaths showed that Rule 43 letters were most often issued in relation to staff training, procedures and protocols not being followed, poor documentation, record-keeping and communication.

Communication concerns are highlighted in a number of areas:

- Between different hospital departments or specialties, including referrals for out patient appointments following a stay in hospital or visit to ED.
- Between different staff involved in patient care, including where they change shift.
- With patients and their families.
- With community healthcare providers about follow-up treatment and after the discharge of patients from hospital.

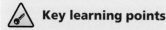 **Key learning points**

**Specific to the case**
- Always take a comprehensive medical history particularly when there is uncertainty. In this case, a travel history was not taken.

**General points**
- Deaths should be discussed with the coroner's officer where the medical practitioner is uncertain about the cause of death
- From April 2013, the role of Medical Examiner will be introduced in England to quality assure the death certification process.

## Reference and further reading

Coroners Statistics 2010, Statistics Bulletin, Ministry of Justice. http://www.justice.gov.uk/downloads/statistics/mojstats/coroners-bulletin-2010.pdf [last accessed 01 June 2012].

Department of Health (2011) Death Certification Reforms: New Duty on Local Authorities. http://www.dh.gov.uk/prod_consum_dh/groups/dh_digitalassets/documents/digitalasset/dh_129894.pdf [last accessed 01 June 2012].

# Case 14 Falling standards

Mrs Owen is a 79-year-old lady who is partially sighted (macular degeneration), has mild to moderate Alzheimer's disease, stable heart failure and osteoarthritis of her knees. She lives in an annexe at her daughter's house and manages to walk short distances within the home but is too unsteady to go out without a lot of assistance. Her daughter takes her shopping once a week in a wheelchair.

Mrs Owen is admitted to hospital with acute delirium resulting from cellulitis of her left leg. She has fallen twice at home in the last 24 hours but without sustaining serious injury. She is seen by a core medical trainee, Dr Manek, who undertakes a thorough assessment and initiates treatment with intravenous flucloxacillin and prophylactic low molecular weight heparin in keeping with local hospital guidelines.

## Are there any other areas that Dr Manek should pay attention to?

Mrs Owen's usual medication is:
Ramipril 5 mg od
Furosemide 40 mg od
Bisoprolol 2.5 mg od
Citalopram 20 mg od
Donepezil 10 mg od
Aspirin 75 mg od
Paracetamol 1.0 gm qds prn.

The staff nurse looking after Mrs Owen tells Dr Manek she is concerned that Mrs Owen is at particularly high risk for falling in hospital and fills out the STRATIFY falls risk assessment tool which she files in the notes. Mrs Owen scores 5/5 on this simple screening tool and so a falls prevention checklist and action plan is completed. Despite being identified as a high risk for falling, Mrs Owen is given a bed in the furthest bay away from the nursing station and although a low bed is advised, none is immediately available. That night, unwitnessed, Mrs Owen gets herself out of bed without asking for help. Predictably, she falls and hits her head on a radiator.

The cover FY1 doctor is asked to review Mrs Owen and he decides the small laceration on her occiput does not require sutures. He reads the notes and concludes she is no more confused than on admission and so takes no further action. The next morning Mrs Owen remains in bed and has to be woken up for breakfast. She seems withdrawn and not at all agitated and perhaps because she is less demanding than on the previous day, the nurse looking after her enters in the notes 'much more settled today'. The Consultant on-take sees Mrs Owen on the ward round but as he has not met her before he too fails to register that reluctance to get out of bed is unusual for her. The cellulitis is already better and the intravenous flucloxacillin is changed to oral and discharge home within the next 48h is anticipated.

## Do you have any concerns about this plan?

Overnight Mrs Owen poses no problems for the nursing staff and she makes no attempt to get up. By the next morning she is very difficult to rouse and Dr Manek suspects she may have sustained a more significant head injury than was initially suspected. An urgent CT scan is arranged which shows a large acute subdural haemorrhage and evidence of a significant mass effect. The regional neurosurgical team is consulted but Mrs Owen's conscious level falls further and a decision is made not to transfer her for neurosurgery. Three days later she dies without regaining consciousness.

## Expert opinion

An internal clinical incident investigation is carried out and the following concerns are raised:
- Although an appropriate assessment of Mrs Owen's risk of falling was made, no action was taken to address the risk.

---

*Avoiding Errors in Adult Medicine*, First Edition. Ian P. Reckless, D. John M. Reynolds, Sally Newman, Joseph E. Raine, Kate Williams and Jonathan Bonser.
© 2013 John Wiley & Sons, Ltd. Published 2013 by John Wiley & Sons, Ltd.

- After the fall occurred no neurological observations were undertaken to chart and identify the falling level of consciousness.
- Staff failed to realize that Mrs Owen's passivity after the fall was symptomatic of a serious underlying problem.
- The late identification of the subdural haemorrhage meant that it was too late to intervene.

This was a preventable death where despite flagging up the risk, no effective measures were put in place. Mrs Owen's daughter also wrote to ask why her mother had been allowed to fall and the hospital acknowledged its shortcomings and stated it would put in place additional education for all staff to highlight the importance of not just making an assessment of risk but also putting in place appropriate measures to mitigate that risk.

### ⚖ Legal comment

Maintaining accurate clinical documentation as a permanent record of the care provided to a patient is a legal duty. Not only does good documentation ensure a written permanent account of the care provided, it also enables for care plans to be communicated between members of the medical and nursing team and with other members of the multi-disciplinary team.

If the Trust has a protocol and staff have taken steps to document the elevated falls risk, but then failed to undertake practical steps to reduce the risk to the patient, this is something of an own goal. Written evidence-based protocols are to be encouraged, but they must be realistic and achievable or else staff are set up to fail. From the defensibility perspective, the Trust may have been better off without a formal falls risk assessment policy.

The complete absence or paucity of documentation is often a key factor in the assessment of defensibility of a potential claim. To a third party, a lack of information implies the worst. Whereas in reality steps may have been taken to observe a patient (such as Mrs Owens in the account above), if it is not documented in the healthcare records then the courts are able to take the view on the balance of probability the care was not provided and no actions were taken.

The preventable death will be reported to the coroner. Depending upon his views of the factual evidence he may return an accidental death verdict. However, given the findings of the internal investigation that no steps were taken to implement the appropriate care plan as a following on from the falls risk assessment and the documented lack of neurological observations, he is more likely to consider a narrative verdict perhaps with a neglect rider. It is good practice to share the SIRI report with both the family and the coroner prior to the inquest hearing.

The modest damages that would be awarded if breach of duty and causation are proved on the balance of probability would be based on the pain and suffering experienced by Mrs Owen after her fall on the ward until she became unconscious and was subsequently unaware of her condition, in addition to the statutory bereavement award, currently set at £11 800.

### ⚠ Key learning points

**General point**
- It is counterproductive for hospitals to have over-ambitious policies and procedures – it is more important for them to have pragmatic policies and procedures and have evidence of compliance with them. A falls policy and procedure is achievable, but it is not realistic to expect that all falls in hospital are preventable.

### Reference

Oliver D, Britton M, Seed P, *et al.* (1997) Development and evaluation of evidence based risk assessment tool (STRATIFY) to predict which elderly inpatients will fall: case control and cohort studies. *Br Med J* 315: 1049–53.

# Section 3: An approach to complaints

# Case 15 A woman with chest pain

Mrs Wilkinson, a 78-year-old widow, presents to the Emergency Department at 5.30 on a Tuesday morning with a three-hour history of central chest pain accompanied by shortness of breath. The pain was initially extremely severe. She has a history of diffuse coronary disease on a background of diabetes. She says that her cardiologist had informed her that she was for 'medical management'. The chest pain is of a different character to previous episodes – she usually experiences discomfort in the jaw and left arm accompanied by mild nausea, brought on by moderate exercise (70–80 metres on the flat).

She continues to smoke and flew back from a three week Caribbean cruise four days ago.

On examination, Mrs Wilkinson continues to have some central chest discomfort and an ache between her shoulders. The pain has reduced in intensity since its onset. Her vital signs demonstrate a tachycardia (130 irregular), tachypnoea of 24 breaths per minute and an oxygen saturation of 92% on air. Breath sounds are present throughout the lung fields with no added sounds.

## What would you do now?

Dr Ahmed, an FY2 doctor, applies supplemental oxygen and administers 300 mg aspirin. She requests an electrocardiogram which demonstrates left bundle branch block and atrial fibrillation. She accesses an electronic discharge summary from eight months earlier which attests to an ECG with LBBB pattern and sinus rhythm at that time. A routine panel of blood tests are sent by the nursing staff including a Troponin I. Mrs Wilkinson's pain seems to be settling.

## What is your differential diagnosis?

The FY2's diagnosis is one of Acute Coronary Syndrome precipitated by a tachyarrhythmia. In addition to the aspirin and oxygen, she prescribes single doses of low molecular weight heparin and clopidogrel, and an oral loading dose of digoxin for rate control.

After two hours, she reviews Mrs Wilkinson again. She is now pain free although still short of breath. She has a heart rate of 110 per minute (AF) and oxygen saturations of 94% on air. She has been able to mobilize to the toilet and back without any worsening in symptoms. Baseline blood results are now available which are normal apart from a modestly elevated troponin I (0.6 ng/ml). Thyroid function test results will be available in 24 hours. A chest X-ray reveals clear lung fields, a small left pleural effusion and borderline cardiomegaly.

## What would you do now?

Dr Ahmed talks on the telephone to the Cardiology Registrar who agrees that this ischaemic episode may have been rate-related and confirms that Mrs Wilkinson has severe multi-vessel disease with poor distal vessels: she is a candidate for neither angiographic nor surgical intervention.

Dr Ahmed remains comfortable with her diagnosis and given that the tachycardia seems to be responding to digoxin and the chest pain has resolved, she decides to discharge Mrs Wilkinson with digoxin (a further loading dose followed by a maintenance dose) and advice to see her GP on Thursday that week for review and results of her thyroid function tests.

On Thursday morning, Mrs Wilkinson fails to attend her GP appointment. After morning surgery, the GP asks the district nurse to make contact with Mrs Wilkinson as she is usually very reliable. The district nurse is unable to contact Mrs Wilkinson by telephone and makes a home visit. She is able to see Mrs Wilkinson on the floor through the sitting room window. The police are called to gain entry to the house and Mrs Wilkinson is confirmed dead.

---

*Avoiding Errors in Adult Medicine*, First Edition. Ian P. Reckless, D. John M. Reynolds, Sally Newman, Joseph E. Raine, Kate Williams and Jonathan Bonser.
© 2013 John Wiley & Sons, Ltd. Published 2013 by John Wiley & Sons, Ltd.

A coroner's post-mortem examination reveals a type B dissection of the aorta which has ruptured intra-thoracically.

Mrs Wilkinson's son is concerned that his mother had been discharged from the Emergency Department within 24 hours of her death and he writes to the hospital seeking an explanation.

## What approach should the clinical director take when responding to this letter?

### ⚠️ Expert opinion

An elevation in serum troponin is not 100% specific for myocardial infarction due to coronary disease. In the case described, misdiagnosis was driven by the assumption that the troponin rise was driven by rate related ischaemia. The history might also have suggested initially a diagnosis of pulmonary embolism and consideration should have been given to performing a CTPA.

Even in the context of the Dr Ahmed's working diagnosis, further errors were made: Dr Ahmed was perhaps lulled in to a false sense of security by the conservative approach advocated by the cardiology registrar, although the registrar's comments were quite focused rather than recommending an overall management plan, and he did not see the patient himself. Even in the absence of interventional options, a patient with myocardial damage regardless of cause would typically be observed in hospital for 24–48 hours. This course of action – appropriate on the basis of the Dr Ahmed's working diagnosis – may have prevented Mrs Wilkinson's death and offered further opportunities to reach the correct diagnosis.

There were a number of clues in Mrs Wilkinson's history that this was not simple acute coronary syndrome – the character and initial severity of the pain, and the presence of a pleural effusion.

### ⚖️ Legal comment

Mrs Wilkinson's son has written a letter of complaint; he is not currently seeking any form of recompense. A complaint response should be sent in line with the formal *NHS Complaints Process*. Using the Department of Health's complaint grading matrix, this letter is likely to be graded as a serious (red) complaint. In accordance with the *Being Open and Honest NHS Policy* the Clinical Director's response should be exactly that.

The patient's death also triggered the Serious Incident Requiring Investigation (SIRI) process by the NHS Trust, with an action plan and final report to be shared with the family.

Mrs Wilkinson's death within 24 hours of discharge from hospital required a referral to the coroner, from which the coroner's post-mortem followed. The coroner's officer liaised with the Trust's legal team in order to obtain a copy of the healthcare records and statements from Trust staff to assist the coroner establish cause of death. Where, as in this case, there has been an SIRI investigation, the report is shared with the coroner as evidence of organizational learning. Where the coroner has significant concerns about patient safety, he has it in his power to write a Rule 43 Letter to the Chief Executive of the Trust (with a copy to the Ministry of Justice) requesting specific reassurance that steps have been taken that would assist to prevent a similar fatality in the future.

Mrs Wilkinson's son would have three years from her date of death to bring a clinical negligence claim (under the 'primary limitation period'). Whilst breach of duty may be established, for the deceased's estate to make a claim for damages under the Law Reform (Miscellaneous) Provisions Act 1934, or any dependents to make a claim under the Fatal Accidents Act 1976, they will also need to establish causation, i.e. would require that the actions or omissions of healthcare professionals had directly resulted in Mrs Wilkinson's death. The coroner's verdict may give greater clarification of the factual cause of death (although the coroner can make no assessment of liability).

If following the coroner's Inquest hearing and response under the complaints process, Mrs Wilkinson's son decides to bring legal action, the Trust would have to notify the NHS Litigation Authority under the Clinical Negligence Scheme for Trusts (CNST) reporting protocol for an evaluation of liability and quantum. There is a litigation risk to the Trust and early expert advice on liability would assist the decision to defend or to reach a settlement. As causation is arguable, this may assist to reach a discounted settlement without an admission of liability. In the absence of a large dependency claim, it is unlikely that the cost benefit analysis of this case would permit it to be run to trial.

If such a legal action was to be brought, it is possible that the NHSLA, the Trust and the individual doctors involved may have differing views on the best form of defence and indeed, whether to actively seek a settlement. For this reason, medical practitioners should make their views known to the Trust's legal team so that these can be considered by the Trust and NHSLA.

---

## Key learning points

### Specific to the case
- A change in the character of chest pain in a patient with angina pectoris requires thorough consideration.
- Troponin is not 100% specific for coronary disease.

### General points
- Care must be taken to avoid being overly selective or extrapolating advice from other clinicians, particularly if provided over the telephone.
- Death within 24 hours of discharge from hospital merits discussion with the coroner's officer for consideration of further action.
- NHS Trusts and individual medical practitioners may have different priorities, motivations and thresholds in relation to defending against a specific clinical negligence claim. For this reason, medical practitioners are encouraged to fully engage with providing their comments and view point to the Trust's legal team.

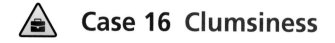

# Case 16 Clumsiness

Mr Stephen Higgins is a 58-year-old partner in an accountancy firm. He is married with two grown-up daughters and a young grandson. He is referred to the neurology outpatient clinic with a history of reduced dexterity and clumsiness in his left hand, present for approximately a month. The referral letter states that Mr Higgins has high blood pressure for which he is taking three antihypertensive agents, and that he smokes. The GP wonders whether the presentation represents a lacunar stroke. Mr Higgins is seen by Dr Miles, an ST5 in neurology.

## What other diagnoses might Dr Miles consider?

Dr Miles takes a thorough history and concludes that the clumsiness was first noted by Mr Higgins some three months ago and that it has progressed a little over that time. On direct questioning, Mr Higgins describes his left leg as feeling somewhat heavy although he has not had any problems getting around – aside from a single fall in the garden a week before the appointment. There are no sensory symptoms. There has been no weight loss, cough or shortness of breath. Examination reveals a left arm that is weaker than the right – the difference more than one might expect on the basis of hand dominance. There appears to be some wasting of the intrinsic muscles of the hand. Reflexes are difficult to elicit. On examination of the lower limbs, reflexes are generally brisk. There is no wasting but there is occasional fasciculation over the anterior thigh. Cranial nerves are entirely normal. Chest examination is normal.

## What is you differential diagnosis at this point?

Dr Miles explains to Mr Higgins that the differential is broad. The most likely diagnosis is a radiculopathy secondary to cervical myelopathy. However, a space occupying lesion or a stroke is possible, and there is a very

small chance of a primary degenerative condition such as motor neurone disease. Dr Miles tells Mr Higgins that he will organize a chest radiograph, a CT scan of the brain and neurophysiological tests in the first instance before reviewing Mr Higgins in the clinic in 4 weeks.

When Mr Higgins returns to clinic 4 weeks later, Dr Miles is on annual leave and he is seen by Dr Wainwright, a clinical research fellow. In a busy clinic, Dr Wainwright reviews the radiology (normal) and the report of nerve conduction studies done a week before (normal conduction velocities and amplitudes). The symptoms have not progressed over this time and Dr Wainwright reassures Mr Higgins that the tests to date have been normal and that the next step is an MRI scan of the cervical spine. Given current symptoms, it is unlikely that a cervical decompression would be appropriate – there is little urgency. He requests this investigation and another appointment is made for 6 months.

## Do you have any comments about the management plan?

Seven months later, Dr Miles once again sees Mr Higgins in the clinic for review. The MRI scan, to Dr Miles' surprise, is entirely normal with no evidence of cervical myelopathy. Mr Higgins states that he has been doing less well. He is no longer able to maintain his garden, a longstanding passion, on account of his increasing clumsiness. He has fallen when climbing up the stairs on two occasions and finds it an effort to get out of the chair. On examination, Mr Higgins' left leg is now wasted. There is clear and widespread fasciculation.

Dr Miles goes back through the records and reviews the nerve conduction studies. He looks at the results of the electromyography (EMG) which appear at the foot of a fax from neurophysiology at the local teaching hospital. He notes that the response of the motor units was said to be 'polyphasic with high amplitude and long duration. Conclusion: consistent . . . ' The remainder of the report is not legible.

*Avoiding Errors in Adult Medicine*, First Edition. Ian P. Reckless, D. John M. Reynolds, Sally Newman, Joseph E. Raine, Kate Williams and Jonathan Bonser.
© 2013 John Wiley & Sons, Ltd. Published 2013 by John Wiley & Sons, Ltd.

Dr Miles explains to Mr Higgins that he needs to revisit the diagnosis and that taken together, all the evidence points to amyotrophic lateral sclerosis, a variant of motor neurone disease. Dr Miles takes time to explain the implications of this diagnosis, and with the nurse specialist present, answers Mr Higgins' questions about prognosis.

Mr Higgins dies a year later. His daughter writes to the hospital and complains about the eight-month delay in diagnosis. She states that she and her family feel robbed of good quality time with her father – had he known of the diagnosis, he would have made the best of his situation, spent time getting to know his grandson rather than fretting about work, and done all sorts of things that he has planned to do in retirement. By the time he did know of the diagnosis and prognosis, it was too late.

**How should the hospital respond?**

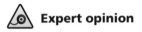 **Expert opinion**

The Neurology Directorate should undertake an investigation into the circumstances surrounding Mr Higgins' treatment. It seems likely that the failure to make an accurate diagnosis on the first opportunity was multifactorial: a partial report from neurophysiology likely due to a defective fax machine; unclear wording on the portion of the EMG report that was communicated; a failure on the part of Dr Wainwright to specifically seek out all the relevant test results; and, a hectic clinic which may not have been reduced in size to accommodate planned leave.

If the hospital is seen to investigate thoroughly, plan and implement improvements, and reduce the chances of a similar event occurring in the future, it is likely that Mr Higgins' family will be satisfied. In this case, putting in place a system by which requested tests are logged and results are followed up, the potential for error could be minimized. Specialist neurophysiologists could also be encouraged to provide a more comprehensive explanation of results, not least as few clinicians will be as au-fait with the interpretation that should be placed on complex – and perhaps normal – measurements.

Many complainants are motivated by a desire to understand what went wrong for them and to prevent others from having the same experience. Relatively few seek financial recompense through a legal process.

**Legal comment**

The daughter's letter of complaint will be responded to under the Trust's complaints policy. This guarantees to acknowledge receipt within three working days and to provide a written response within 25 working days, or longer if agreed by the complainant. The complaints process aims to give a written factual explanation of what treatment the patient has received, to offer an apology for any shortcomings in care and for serious complaints, an action plan to capture any organizational learning that has been identified as necessary as a result of reviewing the complaint.

Local resolution includes the Trust's written letter of response and the offer of a meeting with the patient or patient's family. If a complainant is not satisfied with the Trust's response to their complaint she can refer the matter to the Parliamentary Health Service Ombudsman (PHSO). The PHSO will contact the Trust to establish if local resolution has been completed. If it has not been completed, the PHSO will not review the complaint until it has been. If the Trust confirms that the complaint has been investigated and the Trust has completed local resolution then the PHSO will make an initial review of the Trust's complaints file and the patient's healthcare records to decide whether PHSO investigation is necessary. If the complaint is fully investigated by PHSO then they have recourse to their own independent clinical experts and will report back to the Trust as to whether they uphold the patient's complaint. If the complaint is upheld, the PHSO will make recommendations in its final report for remedy, ranging from a letter of apology from the Chief Executive, to an action plan that demonstrates what steps have been taken to improve systems and procedures to prevent the same events happening to another patient (and family), to an *ex gratia* payment. This latter payment is not compensation, as there is no admission of liability and the payment is made directly by the Trust (and not by the NHSLA) and is designed as a goodwill gesture. The amount is not calculated in accordance with any legal precedent.

**Key learning points**

**General points**
- The clinician who requests an investigation is responsible for ensuring that it is followed up.
- The service providing the diagnostic test should ensure that communication systems are as robust as possible and that the language used in reports is clear and a conclusion is provided.

# Section 4: Competence

# Case 17  A change in plan

Sheila Drake is an 86-year-old lady with cognitive impairment. She is looked after at home by privately-funded 24-hour carers. Mrs Drake had a total anterior circulation stroke a year ago. She is fully dependent and unable to communicate. She is fed a pureed diet by her carers although on occasion, she does not cooperate and appears to be refusing oral intake. She is admitted one evening less responsive than usual. She is seen by Dr Webster, an FY2 doctor in acute medicine.

Dr Webster takes a history from Mrs Drake's carer and examines her. Mrs Drake appears underweight and dehydrated. There is no evidence of sepsis. Dr Webster sends routine bloods and prescribes intravenous fluids. He feels that Mrs Drake ought not to be resuscitated in the event of cardiopulmonary arrest on account of her frailty and comorbidities. The hospital routinely uses a screening tool to identify patients who may require end of life care. Dr Webster considers it likely that Mrs Drake is entering the terminal phase of her life and suggests that the nursing staff ought to have preliminary discussions with Mrs Drake's family when they attend to prepare them for this likely outcome. Following discussion with the duty registrar, a 'Do Not Attempt Resuscitation' (DNAR) form is completed.

## Are you happy with the decisions made by Dr Webster?

An hour or so later, Mrs Margaret De Souza, Mrs Drake's daughter, arrives at the hospital having been informed by the care agency of the admission. She asks to see Dr Webster and be updated on her mother's current situation and the forward care plan.

## Should Dr Webster talk candidly to Mrs De Souza?

Dr Webster explains his findings to Mrs De Souza and updates her on the results of baseline blood tests (which were unremarkable aside from a mild degree of acute renal failure and a reduced serum albumin). He explains the plan to provide intravenous rehydration overnight and outlines the decision that has been made in relation to resuscitation.

Mrs De Souza, who was initially friendly and positive, reacts badly when the issue of resuscitation is raised. Her body language and demeanour changes. Mrs De Souza states that her mother must be resuscitated and that she and her husband, a lawyer, have spoken with the hospital about this on previous occasions. As the conversation continues, Mrs De Souza asserts that Mrs Drake should be given antibiotics in case her deterioration is related to occult infection and she feels that nasogastric feeding would also be appropriate.

## How should Dr Webster react to these requests?

Dr Webster is somewhat taken aback by Mrs De Souza's position and the rather aggressive manner in which she has expressed herself. He states that he will discuss her case with his seniors, and pass on the requests that she has made. However, he notes that the treatment plan will be developed in Mrs Drake's best interests, as perceived by the medical team. Dr Webster explains that Mrs Drake is unable to participate in the decision making process and that nobody is able to direct treatment on behalf of another adult.

At this point, Mrs De Souza tells Dr Webster that she has an enduring power of attorney and as such, she has the necessary authority to direct the treatment that Mrs Drake should have. She produces a letter from a solicitor that appears to confirm that an enduring power of attorney is indeed in place.

## What should Dr Webster do at this point?

Dr Webster reconsiders his treatment plan in the light of the letter. He asks the staff nurse to commence

---

*Avoiding Errors in Adult Medicine*, First Edition. Ian P. Reckless, D. John M. Reynolds, Sally Newman, Joseph E. Raine, Kate Williams and Jonathan Bonser.
© 2013 John Wiley & Sons, Ltd. Published 2013 by John Wiley & Sons, Ltd.

broad spectrum antibiotics and to insert a nasogastric feeding tube. He tells Mrs De Souza that Mrs Drake's resuscitation status will be reviewed with the consultant the following morning but that in the meantime, she will be actively managed if she was to deteriorate.

## ⚠ Expert opinion

This is a challenging situation. In the minds of most people, professional and lay alike, Mrs Drake's existence will be viewed as pretty miserable. From the history given, she had a debilitating and progressive illness prior to her major stroke a year ago and her life experience seems to have deteriorated markedly following that stroke. Many people would argue that her care should be organized to optimize her comfort and dignity, rather than to prolong her life. If despite rehydration, Mrs Drake's condition worsens and she has a cardiac arrest, her weak condition means she is highly unlikely to be resuscitated successfully or without suffering further neurological impairment.

Mrs Drake's daughter, for whatever reason, views things differently and is adamant that all efforts must be made to prolong her mother's life. Dr Webster's initial stance was appropriate – decisions should be made that are consistent with Mrs Drake's best interests. An approach including a baseline assessment, intravenous fluids and good-quality nursing care pending review the next day was both pragmatic and ethically sound. Resuscitation in this context does not seem to be in the best interests of the patient and in any case, it is unlikely that an intensive care team would wish to ventilate Mrs Drake. The line taken by Dr Webster with Mrs De Souza was well reasoned and although it is always preferable to have such discussions once the passage of time has allowed a therapeutic relationship to develop, Mrs De Souza clearly pushed for these discussions to take place at an early stage.

Mrs De Souza told Dr Webster that she had an enduring power of attorney and that this gave her the right to dictate treatment. This is not the case. It is unclear whether Mrs De Souza genuinely believed this to be the situation or whether she wilfully misled Dr Webster in order to achieve the outcome she desired.

Prior to the introduction of the Mental Capacity Act 2005, an Enduring Power of Attorney (EPA) was the mechanism for setting out in advance what a patient wished to happen in the future when they no longer had capacity with regards to his/her property and financial matters.

The Mental Capacity Act 2005 introduced two new types of Lasting Power of Attorney instead of the EPA. These can now cover issues relating to personal welfare (including healthcare) and property and financial affairs. It is no longer possible to establish a new Enduring Power of Attorney although those put in place prior to 2007 remain valid.

It is important to note that even when a Lasting Power of Attorney concerning healthcare is in place, the attorney cannot direct treatment to any greater extent than a competent adult could direct their own management: a specific intervention must always have an appropriate medical indication.

In specific circumstances, where an adult patient has no family or friends who it is appropriate to consult and no attorney (under a registered LPA) to act on their behalf (and have been assessed as lacking capacity to make a necessary decision about serious medical treatment) then the Mental Capacity Act introduces a duty on the NHS to instruct an Independent Mental Capacity Advocate (IMCA). The IMCA will be instructed by the healthcare professional, usually the consultant in charge of care, who will have to make the final decision about whether the proposed serious medical treatment is in the patient's best interests.

The duties of an IMCA are to support the person who lacks capacity and represent their views and interests to the 'decision-maker' (consultant in charge of care); obtain and evaluate information (through interviewing the patient, by examining relevant healthcare records and documents, obtaining the views of professional and paid workers providing care or treatment to the patient, obtain a further medical opinion if required) and prepare a report that the 'decision-maker' (consultant in charge of care) must consider.

The IMCA is not a decision-maker for the person who lacks capacity. They are there to support and represent that person and to ensure that decision-making for the person who lacks capacity is done appropriately in accordance with the MCA.

The only exception to involving an IMCA is where an urgent decision is needed for example to provide emergency life saving treatment. When there is frank disagreement between a patient's next of kin and the medical team then the MCA Code of Practice for healthcare professionals (5.63–5.64) states that any dispute about the best interests of a person who lacks capacity should be resolved, wherever possible, in a quick and cost effective manner. Alternative solutions to disputes, such as informal resolution, formal complaints resolution and mediation should be considered, where appropriate, before an application to the Court of Protection.

## ⚠ Legal comment

No patient, or relative of a patient, can require a particular type of treatment from the healthcare team. All treatment must be clinically indicated and to be in the best interests of the patient. Ideally, the deterioration in a patient's condition necessitating consideration of a DNAR order and the rationale behind the clinical decision-making process which has been undertaken to reach the view that it would not be in a patient's best interests to resuscitate should be communicated to the family in advance of the order being implemented.

The Mental Capacity Act 2005 (MCA) introduced LPAs to encourage patients to plan ahead and to discuss with their next of kin and their family what future care options they would wish to pursue should the relevant circumstances arise, and what 'quality of life issues' are particularly important and pertinent for them as individuals. The person named as being given LPA can then discuss the patient's treatment options with the healthcare team as though he/she were the patient.

The welfare LPA is usually written in terms of treatment that a patient has indicated that they do not wish to undergo and does not give the person named as attorney any legal authority for stipulating the treatment that Mrs Drake should have. The person named in the LPA is only authorized to have discussions with the healthcare team about what the patient's wishes would have been, if the patient had capacity and were able to discuss his/her healthcare treatment options in person. In any event, the person named in the LPA has a legal duty at all times to act in accordance with the best interests of the patient.

All LPAs have to be registered with the Office of the Public Guardian. In addition to the solicitor's letter, it would also be advisable to ask to see the actual LPA document and to check for the hologram registration seal. The Office of the Public Guardian can also be contacted and can confirm if indeed they do hold an LPA for a particular patient.

When assessing the best interests of a patient with regard to a particular treatment option, a second opinion from another consultant, who has not previously been involved in the patient's care, can be useful. For example, in assessing whether or not a patient has capacity and in making DNAR decisions.

In the rare cases where the family of a patient (who does not have capacity) disagrees with the treatment plan proposed by the healthcare team, and alternative solutions, for example a multi-disciplinary team best interests meeting, have not resolved the dispute, then the Trust can consider applying to the Court of Protection for a Best Interests Declaration. Namely, requesting that the Court of Protection decide whether the proposed treatment plan is in the patient's best interests and thereby authorize Trust staff to proceed with the treatment (or withdrawal of treatment) without fear of prosecution. Depending on the urgency for the decision/treatment, the treating consultant will be required to write a statement outlining the patient's medical history, current condition and likely prognosis along with proposed treatment options. Sometimes the Judge who is allocated the case will take evidence from the consultant over the telephone. The Court of Protection will appoint the Official Solicitor's Office to act on behalf of the patient and they will obtain expert evidence, if required, as to whether the course of action proposed by the Trust is in the patient's best interests. If the case is brought by the Trust, then the Trust will also be responsible for the Official Solicitor's costs. This is an intense and expensive process.

Where the patient has appointed an attorney, who can be a family member or a friend or a professional such as a lawyer under a registered personal welfare LPA, then the Court of Protection will also ask to hear evidence from the attorney to obtain background information about the patient's wishes and any other useful information that may assist the Court of Protection's decision about the patient's best interests.

Where a best interests declaration is pending from the Court of Protection, the doctors in charge of the patient's care should always continue to treat in the patient's best interests, keeping the patient as stable as possible.

### ⚠ Key learning points

#### Specific to the case

• The patient's daughter was insistent that she wanted 'everything done'. One should not assume a common understanding of the reality of resuscitation between professionals, patients and families.

#### General points

• Lasting Powers of Attorney (LPAs) have to be registered with the Office of the Public Guardian. Doctors should ask to see the actual LPA document (in addition to any official looking letters) and to check for the hologram registration seal. The Office of the Public Guardian can also be contacted for confirmation.

• The person named in the LPA is only authorized to have discussions with the healthcare team about what the patient's wishes would have been, if the patient had capacity and were able to discuss his/her healthcare treatment options in person.

# Case 18  Starving to death

Doris Evans is an 84 year-old lady with a history of rheumatoid arthritis and cognitive impairment. She has been resident in Parkview care home for six years, over which time her level of dependency has gradually increased. Until a couple of months ago, Mrs Evans was able to mobilize with her Zimmer frame approximately 20 metres to get to the residents' lounge and dining room. However, following a particularly bad cold, she has become bedbound. Her oral intake has been much reduced for some weeks and Mrs Evans now exhibits little interest in the world around her.

The nursing home staff ask a GP registrar to see Mrs Evans on his routine round of Parkview as she has begun to suffer skin break down with two areas of pressure damage over the sacrum and the left heel. Her regular GP is on extended leave. The registrar reviews Mrs Evans and assesses the areas of pressure damage. He looks at her Parkview records and notes that there has been no prior discussion as to what she, her GP and her family would wish to do in relation to hospitalization and the intensity of medical intervention. He is unable to contact Mrs Evans' next of kin (her cousin) and elects to send her to the medical take.

Dr Esposito is the medical registrar on-call. He makes a brief medical assessment of Mrs Evans. She is malnourished and mildly dehydrated. She has two areas of early pressure damage (grade 2) as documented by the GP registrar and there is no sign of frank infection. Haemodynamic indices are within the normal range. Mrs Evans is conscious but withdrawn. She appears to have underlying cognitive impairment and is not orientated.

## What course of action should Dr Esposito follow?

Dr Esposito believes that Mrs Evans is extremely frail and that her long term outlook is not good. There is no evidence of an 'acute' medical problem in terms of infection. It seems unlikely that she will die imminently. Mrs Evans has evidence of skin breakdown and in Dr Esposito's view, appropriate nutritional support and fastidious nursing care will be required if this skin breakdown is to be halted.

Dr Esposito arranges for admission. He prescribed VTE prophylaxis and organizes for a fine bore nasogastric feeding tube to be passed and for Mrs Evans to be placed on the unit's emergency nasogastric feeding regime until reviewed by the dietician. She is at liberty to take oral food and fluid should she wish and should her conscious level be sufficient. There does not appear to be a specific neurological issue with swallowing. A pressure relieving mattress is acquired and a nursing care plan completed. Dr Esposito is conscious of the need to strike an appropriate balance in relation to the intensity of investigation. He sees no indication for an intravenous line or radiology assessment and does not order any blood tests. He places Mrs Evans as 'not for resuscitation'.

## What are your thoughts on this plan?

The next morning, Mrs Evans' care plan is in progress and enteral feeding is in place. She seems comfortable and stable although she remains disorientated and withdrawn. Her cousin (Mrs Kempson) arrives and asks to see the doctor. The FY1 doctor on ward cover, Dr Blewitt, attends half an hour later. Mrs Kempson is keen to receive an update from Dr Blewitt but quickly focuses upon the presence of the feeding tube. She states that Mrs Evans had always said that she wanted to die peacefully and that she would not want 'to be kept alive as a vegetable'. She had been consistent in this view for as long as Mrs Kempson could remember, having helped to nurse her own mother following a disabling stroke. Mrs Kempson asks that the artificial feeding be stopped.

## What is your view?

Dr Blewitt feels that it is not his call to stop the feed and is worried that once an intervention such as feeding

*Avoiding Errors in Adult Medicine*, First Edition. Ian P. Reckless, D. John M. Reynolds, Sally Newman, Joseph E. Raine, Kate Williams and Jonathan Bonser.
© 2013 John Wiley & Sons, Ltd. Published 2013 by John Wiley & Sons, Ltd.

has been commenced, it may be unlawful to withdraw it. Moreover, he agrees with the approach taken by Dr Esposito, and ratified by the consultant on the post-take ward round, the day before: Mrs Evans is not competent to participate in the decision, she is not dying imminently, skin breakdown would constitute an unpleasant and undignified death and it is therefore in her best interests – in the absence of a formal advanced directive – to receive nutritional support.

## Do you agree with Dr Blewitt's thought processes?

Dr Blewitt is on ward cover once again 48 hours later, and is called to the ward about Mrs Evans. The nursing staff have found her to be unresponsive. When last seen half an hour prior, all had been stable. All were aware that she was 'not for resuscitation'.

## What would you put down as the cause of death?

Dr Blewitt fills in the death certificate and elects to write 1a dementia and 2 rheumatoid arthritis. Later on that month, the departmental morbidity and mortality (M&M) meeting considers Mrs Evans' notes. It is noticed that no blood tests were undertaken on admission and the team considers that the most likely cause of death was a cardiac arrest secondary to re-feeding syndrome.

## Expert opinion

Had Mrs Evans' regular GP seen her, it might have been decided that her best interests were served by palliation in the care home setting – irrespective of the pressure sores. Given the paucity of information available to the GP registrar, the course of action was reasonable. Her decline sounds as though it was consistent with advancing dementia, although a depressive element was possible. Mrs Evans was let down by a lack of advance care planning.

She was clearly at risk of re-feeding syndrome and it is imperative to ensure that the information required to manage an intervention (enteral feeding) safely is to hand when embarking upon it. It is likely that Mrs Evans was hypokalaemic and that potassium and magnesium replacement might have prevented her death.

Whilst Dr Esposito's decision-making processes were generally sound, the oversight in relation to bloods clearly violates the Trust's enteral feeding policy. Whilst it can be argued that the outcome was not a bad one for

Mrs Evans (given her cousin's comments), the Trust will need to closely examine its processes to ensure that the risk of this sort of incident recurring are minimized.

## Legal comment

### Advance decisions

Under the Mental Capacity Act (MCA) 2005 statutory rules were introduced with clear safeguards to confirm that people may make a decision in advance to refuse treatment if they should lose capacity in the future. It means that whilst a person retains mental capacity, they can make a decision in advance about medical treatment they might not want in the future when they lack capacity. A patient can use an Advance Decision (also called an Advance Directive) to indicate their wish to refuse all or some forms of medical treatment if they lose capacity in the future. A 'living will' is not a legal term.

From October 2007, to be a valid Advance Decision it will need to:

- be made by a person who is 18 or over and has the capacity to make it;
- specify the treatment to be refused (in lay terms);
- specify the circumstances in which this refusal would apply;
- include an express statement that 'the decision stands even if life is at risk';
- not have been made under the influence or harassment of anyone else;
- not have been modified verbally or in writing since it was made;
- include the date the document was written;
- include the person's signature;
- include the signature of the person witnessing the signature, if there is one.

The code of practice provided to healthcare professionals regarding the MCA states that it would be helpful for information about the name and address of the person's GP to be included and for a copy to be lodged with the GP.

The MCA states that an Advance Decision to refuse treatment must refer to a specified treatment(s) that may set out the circumstances when the refusal should apply. A statement that indicates a general desire not to be treated would not constitute an Advance Decision, but an Advance Decision refusing all treatment in any situation (for example, where a person explains that their decision is based on their religious or personal beliefs) may be valid and applicable.

If doctors are alerted to the possibility that a patient might have made an Advance Decision, reasonable efforts such as contacting relatives of the patient and the patient's GP, should be made to establish whether this is the case. Treatment should not be delayed while attempts are made to establish whether an Advance Decision has been made, if the delay would prejudice the patient's health.

Once the healthcare professionals who are considering treatment have been informed verbally of the existence of an Advance Decision or presented with a written Advance Decision, they need to consider:

- whether it is an Advance Decision within the meaning of the MCA;
- whether it is valid;
- whether it is applicable to the treatment.

An Advance Decision to refuse treatment is not valid if the patient has withdrawn it (this does not need to be in writing), or if the patient has done something clearly inconsistent with the Advance Decision.

There are two issues that should be considered in this case. Firstly, although the next of kin should be consulted about the patient's treatment she does not have any legal authority to make decisions on the patient's behalf. There was a failure to establish in advance whilst she had capacity what her end of life care wish was.

It might be very difficult for a treating doctor to be confident that the patient who has said to have made an oral Advance Decision during the course of the conversation with a relative, had the mental capacity to make a decision at the time and was provided with sufficient information to enable an informed decision to be made.

Also it would be difficult to establish whether the person is subject to the undue influence of the relative at the relevant time. Indeed it may be difficult to establish whether the reported conversation took place at all. Disputes about the existence, validity or applicability of an Advance Decision can be referred to the Court of Protection.

## Withdrawal of treatment

The law places withdrawing treatment in the same category as withholding treatment, not in the category of killing. A doctor may withdraw treatment on the same grounds as they may withhold treatment. The law draws a distinction, as examined in the case of Bland (Airedale NHS Trust v Bland (1993) between where a doctor decides not to provide, or not to continue to provide, treatment or care for his patient which could or might prolong life, and where the doctor decides, for example by administering a drug, to actively bring the patient life to an end. Even if the doctor intends the death of a patient by withholding or withdrawing treatment, then it may be lawful to do so in the best interests of the patient. The British Medical Association Guidelines state there is no ethical distinction between withdrawing and withholding treatment.

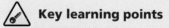 **Key learning points**

### General points

- An Advance Decision (Directive) must contain a number of specified elements in order for it to be considered valid.
- Withholding a treatment and withdrawing that treatment from a patient are similar from ethical and legal standpoints.

# Case 19 An irregular presentation

Mavis Dixon is an 84-year-old lady with advanced dementia, who is admitted from her care home late one Sunday evening. She is reviewed on admission by Dr Ng, the medical FY1 doctor. Mrs Dixon gives no history but seems distressed, shouting out intermittently and being combative with nursing staff when attempts are made to carry out observations or deliver nursing care. The referral letter from the out-of-hours doctor sheds little light on matters (the doctor had never met Mrs Dixon before this evening) and Mrs Dixon's son (her next of kin) is said to be on holiday in India. The care home's background information is sparse in terms of medical history – vascular dementia for seven years, hypertension and atrial fibrillation. Mrs Dixon takes donepezil and no other medications.

## What are your thoughts about Mrs Dixon's presentation?

Observations are eventually possible and reveal a blood pressure of 190/80 and a pulse of 120 in atrial fibrillation (AF). Mrs Dixon is apyrexial. Dr Ng tries to examine her but this proves difficult. The chest seems to be clear. There is a murmur consistent with mixed aortic valve disease. The abdomen seems tense but Mrs Dixon resists examination and it is unclear whether there is an element of voluntary guarding.

Dr Ng sends bloods and undertakes a bedside arterial blood gas (ABG) in order to assess baseline haemoglobin and potassium. His working diagnosis is that of urinary tract sepsis. Dr Ng does not think that Mrs Dixon will tolerate either an intravenous or urinary catheter. Intramuscular doses of ceftriaxone and gentamicin are administered. Dr Ng decides that Mrs Dixon ought not to be resuscitated in the event of cardiorespiratory arrest.

## What are your thoughts about Dr Ng's initial management?

Some six hours later, the registrar on duty reviews Mrs Dixon. She remains unwell and agitated. The registrar notes that inflammatory markers are not significantly elevated and questions the working diagnosis of UTI. He telephones the care home and obtains a history of a sudden onset of acute on chronic confusion associated with apparent abdominal pain (Mrs Dixon had been holding her tummy) and two subsequent episodes of loose blood-stained stool.

## What is the likely diagnosis?

The registrar further reviews Dr Ng's notes and happens across the ABG result which had shown a haemoglobin of 12.8 g/dl and a potassium of 4.3 mmol. The gas also demonstrated a pH of 7.28 and a lactate of 7.6 mmol. The registrar quickly makes a diagnosis of ischaemic bowel but Mrs Dixon's nurse shouts over to him that she has become unresponsive. The registrar assesses Mrs Dixon who has lost her cardiac output. He concurs with Dr Ng's earlier decision not to perform CPR.

The hospital receives a letter from Mrs Dixon's son asking how his mother was allowed to die: if she had been diagnosed earlier, would an operation have saved her; and, who made the decision not to resuscitate her and how could they make this decision without reference to her next of kin?

## How should the service manager for medicine respond?

## Expert opinion

It is likely that the outcome could not have been altered in this case as many surgeons and intensivists would not consider emergency laparotomy as being in such a patient's best interests, given her significant comorbidity. It seems likely that Mrs Dixon's son, given his concerns about the resuscitation decision, may think otherwise. However, both decisions – the appropriateness of laparotomy and resuscitation – lie with the professional who might undertake them. With any patient

*Avoiding Errors in Adult Medicine*, First Edition. Ian P. Reckless, D. John M. Reynolds, Sally Newman, Joseph E. Raine, Kate Williams and Jonathan Bonser.
© 2013 John Wiley & Sons, Ltd. Published 2013 by John Wiley & Sons, Ltd.

intervention, the professional must be of the view that an intervention may offer the patient benefit (and therefore be in the patient's interests) and, where the patient is competent, the patient must also consent to the intervention before it can be carried out. If the professional does not consider an intervention to be of potential benefit, then a patient (or their representative) cannot force the professional's hand into undertaking the intervention.

In this particular case, Mrs Dixon's diagnosis could have been made a few hours earlier had further efforts been made to obtain a more thorough history. It is difficult for the Trust to defend a situation where a registered doctor had not assessed a patient within six hours of arrival, and where a resuscitation decision is made by a pre-registration doctor without reference to senior colleagues.

The Trust should apologize for the shortcomings in Mrs Dixon's care but be clear about how decisions about resuscitation and other interventions are made.

## Legal comment

It is important that junior doctors are able to escalate decisions with regard to CPR to a more senior colleague in a timely fashion. There is likely to be a Trust protocol or guideline with regard to Do Not Attempt Resuscitation (DNAR) orders outlining the steps that must be taken and the staff who should be involved in the approval of a DNAR order. The Trust is also vulnerable in its position, as there appears to be no documented assessment of the patient's capacity prior to a best interests decision. It is important at all times, particularly towards the end of life, that decisions as significant as this one are communicated with the next of kin in advance of an emergency situation arising.

## Key learning points

### Specific to the case
• DNAR decision-making has a high profile and should be handled with particular care.
• Trust guidelines will specify the appropriate seniority for decision makers and the timelines for senior review.

### General points
• Decisions that are made in the best interests of a patient lacking in competence should be clearly documented.
• Such decisions should be made, where possible, following discussion with the patient's next of kin and other advocates.
• Key decisions made in relation to a patient's care should be communicated to the patient and the patient's advocate in a timely fashion (whether or not the patient or advocate agrees with those decisions).

## Further reading

General Medical Council (2010) Treatment and care towards the end of life: good practice in decision making. http://www.gmc-uk.org/static/documents/content/End_of_life.pdf [last accessed 01 June 2012].

# Case 20 Irrational but not incompetent

Peter Walton is a 57-year-old sales representative who develops unsteadiness when walking and a persistent frontal headache on Friday morning. His wife is worried about him but he refuses to see a GP as he has had a lifelong antipathy to medical and dental interventions – in fact he has never registered at a practice. He heads off to work but is involved in a minor road traffic accident when he fails to notice a vehicle pulling out to pass him in a queue of cars. An ambulance is called and although they confirm that no one has significant injury, they do note that Mr Walton's blood pressure is 266/153 and they persuade him to go to the local emergency department.

Dr Goldberg is the staff grade on duty and he finds Mr Walton to be very dismissive and apparently irritated by having been brought to hospital. Over the next 90 minutes, Mr Walton's blood pressure remains very high and Dr Goldberg is concerned that this level of hypertension is causing the headache, unsteadiness and may well have contributed to the accident. Mr Walton agrees to have some blood tests, a chest X-ray and ECG but is very clear he will not be staying in hospital and wishes to go.

The ECG shows left ventricular hypertrophy with strain and there is cardiomegaly on the chest X-ray. Mr Walton has a potassium of 3.2 mmol/l and a creatinine of 165 mmol/l. Dr Goldberg tells Mr Walton that he believes that his recent symptoms are all a result of severe hypertension and that left untreated the risk of serious complications like stroke or death are high. This is dismissed by the patient who says 'your blood pressure would be high if you'd just had an accident and had been forced to come in to hospital against your will – there's nothing wrong with me that a bit of rest won't cure'. By now, Mrs Walton has arrived and she tries to persuade her husband to stay while Dr Goldberg does more investigations and starts some treatment, but he is very brusque with her and demands to be taken home.

## What should Dr Goldberg do at this point?

5 mg amlodipine is prescribed, but Mr Walton refuses it and so Dr Goldberg calls the medical consultant on take for advice on how to proceed. Dr Mason arrives and agrees with the clinical findings and the likely diagnosis of hypertensive emergency. He too explains the risks to Mr Walton of not staring immediate treatment, and he wonders if Mr Walton's judgement is clouded by hypertensive encephalopathy.

## How would you assess Mr Walton's competence to make a decision about his care?

Dr Mason considers that Mr Walton appears to be able to retain the information given to him and he appears to be able to reiterate the consequences of no treatment, including the risk of death. He however denies that this is as serious as the medical team are making out and he asserts he will take his own discharge against medical advice. Reluctantly Dr Mason accepts this and documents the conversation he has had in the notes. He provides Mr Walton with an appointment to return to clinic the next day and urges him to register with a GP as soon as possible. He also provides Mr Walton with a supply of amlodipine tablets and instructions on how to take them if he should change his mind. Mrs Walton is very upset but defers to her husband's decision and they leave the department.

## Do you agree with Dr Mason's course of action?

Two days later Mr Walton is readmitted as an emergency in status epilepticus. His blood pressure is initially unrecordably high. He is given intravenous diazepam and phenytoin and a CT scan of his head is performed which shows a large posterior fossa intracerebral

*Avoiding Errors in Adult Medicine*, First Edition. Ian P. Reckless, D. John M. Reynolds, Sally Newman, Joseph E. Raine, Kate Williams and Jonathan Bonser.
© 2013 John Wiley & Sons, Ltd. Published 2013 by John Wiley & Sons, Ltd.

haemorrhage. Despite obtaining control of the blood pressure gradually over the next six hours, he does not regain consciousness and dies later that day.

Mr Walton's son, who is a psychiatric nurse, had been at his father's bedside for the last few hours of his life and he is very angry with the medical team. He asserts that they failed to insist he received treatment two days earlier that would have saved his life. He also says he believes his father's decision was entirely out of character and was symptomatic of impaired cognition due to the severity of the hypertension and he should have been detained and treated under 'common law'.

### Expert opinion

This case was very difficult. Mr Walton had evidence that his hypertension was causing neurological impairment (headache, unsteadiness, lack of awareness when driving, irritability) and yet he was able to answer the rather basic questions which were used in the assessment of competence. Mrs Walton was frightened of her husband and did not feel she could push him further to comply. The son later expressed the opinion that this was out of character for his father and evidence that he was not thinking normally.

Dr Mason discusses the case with the Trust Medical Director and with his defence union, and in due course a complaint is made by the son against both Dr Mason and Dr Goldberg to the General Medical Council.

### Legal comment

Mental capacity is decision specific and time specific. Can the person make this decision as this time? The five principles of the Mental Capacity Act (MCA) 2005 are:
- Presume capacity unless there is evidence otherwise.
- Do all you can to maximize a person's capacity.
- Unwise or eccentric decisions don't of themselves prove lack of capacity.
- If you are making a decision for or about someone who lacking capacity; always act in the best interests of the person.
- In making a best interest decision, seek the least restrictive option that will meet the person's needs.

Assessing capacity is a two-stage process. Does the person have an impairment of mind or brain, or is there some sort of disturbance affecting the way their mind or brain works, either on a temporary on permanent basis? If so, does that impairment or disturbance mean that the

person is unable to make the decision in question at the time that it needs to be made?

A person has capacity to make a particular decision only if they can carry out all four of these following steps:
1. understand appropriately presented information about that decision;
2. retain the information for long enough to:
3. use and weigh it to make a decision; and
4. communicate the decision by any recognizable means.

Since the introduction of the MCA there is no such thing as 'detention under common law'. The MCA and DOLS (Deprivation of Liberty Safeguards) allow use of least restrictive restraint to permit treatment in the best interests of the patient until capacity is regained. A patient with capacity has the right to reject all reasonable suggested clinical treatment options and to follow the option of no clinical treatment. This arises from the principle of patient autonomy and is now enshrined in the five key principles of the MCA.

Many Trusts have a self-discharge form which asks the patient to sign and date a form which indicates that the advice of the treating doctor is for the patient to remain in hospital but that the patient has capacity and wishes to self-discharge home despite the clinical advice in his/her best interests.

It is advisable to document in the patient's healthcare records what information has been given, either by way of patient information leaflet or verbal instruction about adverse symptoms to be alert for and how/who to contact if the patient's condition deteriorates and he/she starts to show signs of these symptoms.

### Key learning points

**General points**
- Capacity must be determined in conjunction with the principles outlined in the Mental Capacity Act 2005.
- Severe hypertension of the magnitude seen in Mr Walton's case is becoming unusual as a result of primary care screening and better management of hypertension. However many middle aged men still avoid health screening and they are a group at particular risk. Untreated severe hypertension carries a mortality in excess of 75% at one year and the common causes of death are stroke and heart failure.

# Section 5: Restraint

# Case 21  A challenging discharge

Mr Stanislavski is a 63-year-old former alcoholic who was admitted to the Acute Medical Unit (AMU) following an unwitnessed collapse at his care home. He has poor short-term memory and had been unable to provide detailed information on the circumstances of the event. He has no close family. Following 24 hours of observation (including cardiac monitoring), no firm diagnosis has been made and Mr Stanislavski appears well in himself. He is ambulant.

Mr Stanislavski underwent a quadruple coronary bypass two years ago and is on appropriate medications for the secondary prevention of arterial disease.

## What would you do?

Dr Pirelli, the CT2 attached to the team, sees Mr Stanislavski and explains to him that no injuries have resulted from his collapse and that there is no evidence of any sinister cause for the episode. Dr Pirelli therefore recommends discharge from the hospital. Mr Stanislavski is pleased to be able to leave the AMU.

Whilst Dr Pirelli is preparing the patient's discharge paperwork, the staff nurse approaches him and states that Mr Stanislavski is refusing to return to his care home. When Dr Pirelli talks to him about this, he alleges that the staff there are unpleasant to him, that the environment is dirty and that he is not permitted to have any visitors. Mr Stanislavski says that he is in the process of complaining to the local council about his treatment.

## How would you manage the situation?

Dr Pirelli telephones the care home to speak to a staff member about the background. He is unable to speak to the manager but one of the carers explains that Mr Stanislavski is often difficult when he attends hospital but that he quickly settles into a normal routine when

back at the care home. Mr Stanislavski has few visitors but this is because he has few friends rather than on account of any action on the part of the care home. Dr Pirelli and the staff nurse tell Mr Stanislavski that he must return to the care home. He becomes agitated and aggressive and begins to pace up and down looking for the exit. He pushes a healthcare assistant who he says is obstructing his way.

## What would you do now?

Dr Pirelli telephones the consultant who is of the view that Mr Stanislavski is not competent to take his own discharge and that he should be held in his best interests until the situation can be clarified with the care home manager, the duty social worker and any other relevant parties. The nursing staff call hospital security but on arrival they state that they are not permitted to restrain Mr Stanislavski.

## What do you think about the position of the hospital security team?

The consultant comes to the AMU and documents that Mr Stanislavski should be prevented from leaving the hospital until such a time as matters can be clarified. She then examines Mr Stanislavski's lengthy medical notes in detail. The notes describe a protracted discharge process (six months) following the coronary bypass procedure at which time Mr Stanislavski's memory problems had become evident. He had been seen extensively by neurologists and psychologists at that time and had been judged incapable of living independently. A past history of alcoholism and impulsive gambling was also described. Ultimately, he had been forced to reside in a care home against his expressed wishes under the terms of a 'Deprivation of Liberty order', supervised by the local authority. The consultant telephones the local authority's responsible officer and confirms that the DOL order remains in place.

*Avoiding Errors in Adult Medicine*, First Edition. Ian P. Reckless, D. John M. Reynolds, Sally Newman, Joseph E. Raine, Kate Williams and Jonathan Bonser.
© 2013 John Wiley & Sons, Ltd. Published 2013 by John Wiley & Sons, Ltd.

Following confirmation, the consultant explains to Mr Stanislavski that he will be returning to the care home with or without assistance from the police. She explains also that Mr Stanislavski's care manager will make contact with him later in the week to discuss his concerns about the care home once again. Mr Stanislavski returns quietly to the care home with an ambulance escort.

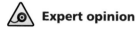

## Expert opinion

The key issues in this case relate to competence and the various legal mechanisms that may be in operation when a person is deprived of their liberty. Clinicians tend to have experience of patients detained in custody (police or prison service) or detained under the Mental Health Act 1983 but the Deprivation of Liberty safeguards are new under the Mental Capacity Act 2005. In Mr Stanislavski's case, careful examination of the medical records quickly provided the necessary background information. However, the case highlights the importance of clear and appropriate communication between carers in hospital and the community.

In this case, the team was able to assure itself that the care home was a safe discharge destination following discussion with the local authority's responsible officer. It was reasonable to ask hospital security staff to assist in restraining Mr Stanislavski for a proportionate and limited time in his best interests to prevent harm to Mr Stanislavski but it is important that the medical staff should document the request (and the rationale) in the medical notes.

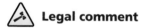

## Legal comment

### Deprivation of Liberty Safeguards (DOLS)

The Mental Capacity Act (MCA) 2005 came into force in October 2007 and provides a statutory framework for acting and making decisions on behalf of individuals who lack the mental capacity to do so themselves. The MCA promotes the involvement of the individual in decision making wherever feasible. It also promotes the involvement of an Independent Mental Capacity Advocate (IMCA) where the individual lacks competence and has no friends and family.

Provisions of the MCA include the Deprivation of Liberty Safeguards (DOLS) that focus on vulnerable people within society who, for their own safety and in their best interests, may need to be accommodated under care and treatment regimes for which they lack the capacity to consent. Such regimes may have the effect of depriving them of their liberty.

Under DOLS, the Managing Authority (a care home or an NHS Trust) must apply to the Supervisory Body (the local authority or PCT respectively) for authorization of Deprivation of Liberty (Standard Authorization). The Managing Authority can authorize itself to deprive an individual of liberty for up to seven days if the need is urgent and where Standard Authorization has been applied for but not yet granted.

The Supervisory Body commissions a series of best interest and medical assessments and either grants or refuses Standard Authorization. The standardized assessments are carried out by specifically trained health or social care professionals (Best Interests Assessors), who cannot be directly involved in the care of the patient, and specially trained doctors with expertise in mental health (Medical Assessors), who can know the patient.

A Managing Authority may also apply for Standard Authorization prior to the deprivation of liberty occurring. This may apply if a person who lacks capacity is about to be admitted to a hospital electively. The Emergency Department (and some assessment areas) may be treated as outside the hospital for the purposes of DOLS when providing urgent and life-saving treatment: an acute NHS Trust will generally only need to apply to the PCT for a DOLS authorization if a patient is admitted as in-patient into the 'hospital proper'. This is because restraint lasting only a matter of hours or a few days for necessary clinical treatment is usually authorized under the Mental Capacity Act (Sections 5 and 6) and does not require formal authorization under the DOLS process.

All hospitals should have a DOLS lead, who will be able to provide advice and assistance in the completion and submission of the appropriate forms to the Supervisory Body.

### Security staff and restraint

Restraint is defined by Section 6 of the Mental Capacity Act 2005 as 'the use or threat of force to help to do an act which the person resists, or the restriction of the person's liberty of movement, whether or not they resist'.

Restraint is legally permissible where it is necessary to protect a person from harm and when it is proportionate to the likelihood and seriousness of that harm. However, the MCA does not allow restraint so intense or long-lasting that it amounts to deprivation of liberty: in such circumstances, restraint must be authorized either through the DOLS process or by the Court of Protection.

Restraint may also be used to administer care or treatment (under section 6 of the MCA) provided it is proportionate and in the person's best interests.

In this case, it would have been reasonable to have used restraint to prevent Mr Stanislavski leaving the hospital premises until the circumstances were clarified. In addition, the existence of a DOLS authorization in the care home (provided Mr Stanislavski was not admitted to a ward, which would immediately cause his DOLS authorization to lapse since authorization is site specific) is regarded as providing evidence that the person's residence in the care home has been robustly assessed as being in his best interests, and such restriction of his freedom as proportionate to the risk and seriousness of harm.

### ⚠ Key learning points

**Specific to the case**

- Allegations of mistreatment should be reported to the lead for vulnerable adults, either within the hospital or in the community.
- The use of restraint in hospital may be appropriate in the management of a patient who lacks capacity to consent to arrangements proposed for his care and/or treatment, as long as it is in his best interests, proportionate to the risk of harm that the patient's behaviour poses to himself, and as long as it represents the least restrictive option to meet the needs of the patient.
- The Deprivation of Liberty Safeguards (DOLS) of the Mental Capacity Act 2005 permit patients who lack competence to be accommodated and treated in a manner contrary to their expressed wishes to receive urgent and life-saving treatment prior to obtaining appropriate formal authorization to continue to deprive them of liberty.

# Case 22  Ruling out the organic

Paul Giardelli is a 20-year-old university student. He is brought to the Emergency Department in the early hours of a Sunday morning by ambulance staff, with a police escort. He had been found walking naked up and down the high street, going into fast food restaurants, taking food from customers and putting it all into the rubbish bins. He had accused staff members of trying to murder the public. There had been an altercation with security staff and Mr Giardelli's face is covered in blood, his nose appears to be broken and he has a scalp laceration.

Mr Giardelli is assessed by an Emergency Department nurse (his blood pressure is stable, he has a tachycardia and a temperature of 37.9 °C) and is seen by the duty F2, Dr El-Sheikh. Mr Giardelli seems withdrawn but when he believes that the attention of the police officers is elsewhere, quickly tells Dr El-Sheikh that the whole town is being poisoned. The supervisor from Mr Giardelli's Hall of Residence attends and tells Dr El-Sheikh that Mr Giardelli is usually a popular and high functioning student. She believes that he and his group of friends use cannabis intermittently. He had been appeared entirely normal when she had seen him 36 hours prior.

## What do you think is going on and how will you investigate Mr Giardelli?

Dr El-Sheikh believes that Mr Giardelli's presentation is that of an acute psychosis, possibly brought on by illicit drug use. He sends a number of blood tests in order to rule out organic pathology. In view of the history of head injury, he elects to undertake a CT scan of the head. On the third attempt, Mr Giardelli is able to cooperate adequately to tolerate the scan. A radiologist views the images remotely and confirms that there is no evidence of extradural, subdural or parenchymal bleeding. There is no skull fracture.

Whilst being transferred back from radiology to the Emergency Department, Mr Giardelli suddenly grabs the porter by his collar and threatens him, saying that he knows he is the ringleader of the poisoning campaign. He pushes the porter into a corner and stares hard at him, breathing heavily before spitting at him. The staff nurse pages security and after a minute or so, two security guards arrive from the departmental coffee room. They take Mr Giardelli down to the floor and restrain him whilst the porter is able to move away from the area. Dr El-Sheikh and the staff nurse are able to calm Mr Giardelli down and he returns of his own accord to the treatment room.

Electrolytes and white count are normal. The CRP is moderately elevated (13mg/l). Dr El-Sheikh sutures the scalp wound and refers Paul on to the inpatient acute psychiatric service with an appointment to return to ENT clinic for assessment of his nasal injuries a week later. One of the security guards remains in the room during treatment. Dr El-Sheikh states in his referral that he believes that Mr Giardelli will need sectioning under the Mental Capacity Act 2005.

## What do you think of this course of action?

Eight hours later, Mr Giardelli is brought back to the Emergency Department from the psychiatric unit (he had been sectioned for assessment). He is in *status epilepticus* and his seizures have not yet responded to diazepam administered by the ambulance staff. Blood glucose is normal. Mr Giardelli is given lorazepam and a phenytoin infusion is commenced. His seizures are continuing fifteen minutes later and ITU attend and sedate, intubate and ventilate Mr Giardelli in order to settle his seizures. A further CT scan is undertaken which shows subtle hypodensity in the temporal lobes.

## What is the likely diagnosis and the appropriate management?

Mr Giardelli is cared for on the intensive care unit. A working diagnosis of viral meningo-encephalitis is

*Avoiding Errors in Adult Medicine*, First Edition. Ian P. Reckless, D. John M. Reynolds, Sally Newman, Joseph E. Raine, Kate Williams and Jonathan Bonser.
© 2013 John Wiley & Sons, Ltd. Published 2013 by John Wiley & Sons, Ltd.

made and Mr Giardelli is commenced on intravenous aciclovir and ceftriaxone (to cover bacterial meningitis) until CSF is obtained and analysed.

CSF is found to contain an excess of lymphocytes and protein is marginally elevated. PCR is subsequently positive for HSV-1. Mr Giardelli receives a ten-day course of aciclovir. He is extubated on day 2 but it is apparent that he has a modest left-sided weakness and there is an early suggestion of neuropsychological deficit.

## Expert opinion

It seems that Dr El-Sheik's assessment of Mr Giardelli may have been overly influenced by the behavioural and forensic aspects of the presentation, and perhaps a desire to progress Mr Giardelli through to a 'more appropriate' venue (acute psychiatric assessment unit) quickly.

In retrospect, the features suggesting encephalitis are obvious – specifically, acute behavioural change, pyrexia and tachycardia. The history of illicit drug use is soft. As a student, Mr Giardelli is in a high risk group in respect of CNS infection. Early CT imaging is insensitive for the diagnosis of encephalitis. A lumbar puncture, whilst doubtless challenging, was indicated upon Mr Giardelli's first presentation. HSV PCR is highly sensitive.

The case also raises questions in relation to the quality of information sharing between staff in the ED (whether or not Dr El-Sheikh was aware of the tachycardia and pyrexia) and the level of support available to junior doctors out of hours.

The hospital will likely be liable for any long-term impact that this episode has on Mr Giardelli – the diagnosis was delayed and earlier diagnosis and intervention may have reduced the extent of parenchymal brain damage and indeed averted the seizures.

Of note, Dr El-Sheikh was mistaken in believing that Mr Giardelli could be sectioned under the Mental Capacity Act 2005 – the Mental Health Act 1983 is the relevant legislation here.

## Legal comment

A clear distinction must be made between the remit of the Mental Health Act 1983 (MHA) and the Mental Capacity Act 2005 (MCA). The MHA legislation is mainly concerned with the compulsory care and treatment of patients with mental health problems. It covers detention in hospital for mental health treatment, supervised community treatment and guardianship. Contrast this with the remit of the MCA legislation which covers decision-making for people who lack capacity to make decisions for themselves or who have capacity and want to make preparations for a future time when they may lack capacity. It sets out who can take decisions, in what situations and how they should go about it. The Deprivation of Liberty Safeguards (DOLs) is a framework of safeguards under the MCA for people who need to be deprived of their liberty in a hospital or a care home in their best interests for care or treatment and who lack the capacity to consent to the arrangements made for their care or treatment.

Section 6 (4) of the MCA states that someone is using restraint if they use force, or threaten to use force, to make someone do something that they are resisting, or restrict a person's freedom of movement, whether they are resisting or not.

However, the MCA recognizes that restraint is appropriate when it is used to prevent harm to a patient who lacks capacity and is a proportionate response to the likelihood of serious harm. Appropriate use of limited, temporary restraint falls short of a deprivation of liberty.

Preventing a person from leaving hospital unaccompanied because there is a risk that they would try to cross a road in a dangerous way, for example, is likely to be seen as a proportionate restriction or restraint to prevent the person from coming to harm. That would be unlikely, in itself, to constitute a deprivation of liberty. Similarly, asking a member of staff to guard a patient against immediate harm is unlikely in itself to amount to a deprivation of liberty.

The European Court of Human Rights has also indicated that the duration of any restriction is a relevant factor when considering whether or not a person is deprived of their liberty. This suggests that actions that are immediately necessary to prevent harm to the patient or to the members of staff may not, in themselves, constitute a deprivation of liberty.

However, where the restriction or restraint is frequent, cumulative and ongoing, or if there are other factors present, then care providers should consider whether this has gone beyond permissible restraint, as defined in the MCA. If so, then they must apply for authorization under the Deprivation of Liberty Safeguards to the Supervisory Authority (Primary Care Trust) or change their care provision to reduce the level of restraint.

In an emergency situation, minimal restraint is permitted to obtain specimens and instigate necessary clinical treatment for a potentially life-threatening condition. As Mr Giardelli's condition deteriorates, he will come to lack capacity and, in accordance with the MCA, the consultant in charge of his care is permitted to act in his best interest. Conversely, as the antiviral regime takes effect, the state of Mr Giardelli's capacity may improve. There will then be a need to monitor his capacity monitor his capacity to contribute to decision-making about his ongoing clinical treatment. The consultant in charge of Mr Giardelli's care should also seek information from his family and friends as to what course of management is in his wider best interests whilst he has impaired capacity.

> ### ⚠ Key learning points
>
> #### Specific to the case
> - Restraint is appropriate when it is proportionate and aimed at reducing the risk of harm to a patient or those around them.
>
> #### General points
> - The Mental Health Act 1983 is concerned with the management of people with mental health problems.
> - The Mental Capacity Act 2005 is concerned with the management of people without mental capacity.
> - Viral encephalitis may present in a way which initially mimics psychosis and it is an important differential diagnosis to consider, particularly if the patient is pyrexial or gives a history of a short prodromal illness.

# Case 23 Endless wandering

Dr Stefan Jacobs is a 92-year-old retired GP. He was admitted to the hospital five days ago having been found by his daughter, visiting from South Africa, to be struggling to manage his own affairs at home. On admission, Dr Jacobs had been unkempt and malnourished. His house had been in quite a state with evidence of vermin infestation. Over a thousand unopened copies of the *British Medical Journal* had been stacked up along one side of the staircase – some of them over 20 years old.

Dr Jacobs's daughter had described him as always having been 'a law unto himself'. People seemed to regard him as a something of a character, although his behaviour had become more unusual and insular over the last 10–15 years since the death of his wife. He has no close friends and no hobbies, having always been fully absorbed in his work. Contact with family has become rare.

Dr Cheung, a consultant gastroenterologist, is popping into his office one Saturday morning to collect some job applications to review at home over the weekend. He meets Dr Jacobs who has wandered off the ward in the lift lobby. Dr Cheung sees Dr Jacobs walking into the lift and notices that his hospital gown (the only thing he is wearing) is undone at the back and that he is carrying all his belongings in a carrier bag along with four copies of the BNF (all labelled as belonging to Mulberry ward). Dr Cheung thinks this is odd and asks the patient (who he has not met before) if he is OK and whether he would like any help. Dr Jacobs replies that he is fine and that he is heading to the tea rooms for a sandwich.

Dr Cheung is worried about Dr Jacobs and persuades him to take a seat in the lift lobby whilst he calls a nurse from Mulberry ward. The nurse arrives and thanks Dr Cheung. She says that this is the sixth occasion on which Dr Jacobs has left the ward since last night and that there aren't enough staff to cope – not least because the ward has two very sick patients. Dr Jacobs had been a nuisance all night – pulling at another patient's catheter bag on one occasion and hiding all the ward files (protocols, procedures, nursing off duty) under his bed. Security had been to the ward several times but had had to return to ED. Half an hour ago, Dr Jacobs had attempted to strike the domestic with his walking stick when he had come to collect his breakfast tray.

## What should Dr Cheung do?

Dr Cheung has every sympathy for the staff nurse, whom he has known for the best part of a decade, and he offers to prescribe a sedative for Dr Jacobs. Dr Jacobs has no wish to take any medicines and Dr Cheung therefore administers 2 mg of lorazepam intramuscularly whilst two staff members hold him down in a chair. Dr Cheung then leaves the ward and proceeds to his office to collect the job applications. Twenty minutes later, Dr Jacobs is much more placid and allows staff to help him to his bed where he sleeps on and off for the remainder of the day.

## Expert opinion

There are two elements to this case which deserve discussion: the safety of the intervention made by Dr Cheung and the ethical and legal aspects of restraint.

It seems that Dr Cheung has acted with the best of intentions. He has found an elderly man who appears to have limited mental capacity attempting to leave the ward in odd circumstances. Dr Cheung was worried about his safety and therefore contacted the ward team to collect the patient. At that point, on hearing of the difficulties faced by the ward team the previous night, Dr Cheung elected to assist them by sedating the patient.

However, it is by no means clear that Dr Cheung weighed up all the relevant factors in relation to the risks and benefits of this course of action. Aside from the

---

*Avoiding Errors in Adult Medicine*, First Edition. Ian P. Reckless, D. John M. Reynolds, Sally Newman, Joseph E. Raine, Kate Williams and Jonathan Bonser.
© 2013 John Wiley & Sons, Ltd. Published 2013 by John Wiley & Sons, Ltd.

prescription there was no documentation at all. Several questions arise:

- Was Dr Jacobs considered to lack capacity?
- What were the perceived dangers to Dr Jacobs and others?
- Was there any less restrictive way of managing the situation?
- Was the choice of drug appropriate?
- Was any effort made to consider relevant comorbidities?
- Was any effort made to assess for precipitants of delirium?
- Was any effort made to ascertain renal function?
- Were appropriate arrangements made for the monitoring of a sedated patient?
- Was the ward team covering that weekend made aware of Dr Cheung's helpful intervention?

From a legal and ethical perspective, it is Dr Cheung's responsibility to ensure that intervention is required and justified, and that the least restrictive course of action is followed. This does not appear to be the case with Dr Jacobs who will be at heightened risk of falls, dehydration, renal failure, respiratory compromise and VTE following the intervention. Furthermore, he will be highly likely to display further challenging behaviour when the lorazepam wears off give that the aetiology has not been addressed.

## ⚠️ Legal comment

Under the Mental Capacity Act (MCA) 2005 it is the role of the 'clinical decision-maker' (the consultant in charge of the patient's care) to make the best interests assessment. It was not appropriate for Dr Cheung to have intervened in this manner.

The more appropriate course of action for Dr Cheung would have been to contact the consultant in charge of the patient's care to notify him of his concerns and permit the treating consultant to act.

The administration of the sedative may have been appropriate if it was the least restrictive method to ensure the safety of the patient and to avoid harm to staff.

## 🔑 Key learning points

### Specific to the case
- Doctors should be cautious of making informal interventions to the care being given by colleagues to patients.

### General points
- Best interests assessments should be made by the consultant with overall responsibility for the care of the patient.
- Restraint, where used, should be the least restrictive form possible applied for as short a period as possible in accordance with the principles of the Mental Capacity Act 2005.

# Case 24  Can you please take these handcuffs off?

Mike Turner is a 61-year-old man who is currently detained in prison at Her Majesty's pleasure. He has been a lifelong smoker (with a 50-pack-year history) and has a strong family history of premature cardiac disease. Over the last few weeks he has noticed exertional chest discomfort which he has put down to indigestion. Today, he develops heavy central chest pain while at rest in his cell and he seeks help from the prison medical officer who decides that he should be assessed in hospital and admission is arranged. Two prison warders accompany Mr Turner, shackled to him by handcuffs and chains.

### What issues will the admitting doctor likely wish to consider?

On arrival in hospital Mr Turner is seen in the Acute Medical Unit by Dr Jenkins who asks the prison officers if she may take a history and examine Mr Turner without them present but they refuse. This seems unsatisfactory to Dr Jenkins and she persists in asking the officers to leave on the grounds of patient privacy and dignity and an argument ensues but the restraints are not removed. Dr Jenkins feels browbeaten and is upset by having failed to convince the prison officers. She wants, amongst other things, to ask Mr Turner about his use of recreational drugs including cocaine but does not feel he would be likely to give a truthful answer in the presence of prison officers. Recording an ECG is made cumbersome by the restraints and she finds inserting a venous cannula difficult and settles for an antecubital site rather than the forearm which would normally have been her preference. On account of nerves, she takes several attempts to insert the line.

Mr Turner's history is consistent with an acute coronary syndrome and his ECG shows inferolateral ST changes. A troponin taken 8 hours after the onset of pain is elevated and coronary angiography is scheduled for the next day. Treatment with aspirin, clopidogrel, low molecular weight heparin, a statin and a beta blocker are all commenced and agreed by the on-take consultant physician. Angiography subsequently demonstrates diffuse coronary disease and a decision is made to manage Mr Turner with medication rather than with coronary artery stenting or surgery in the first instance.

Six weeks after he has been discharged back to prison, the hospital receives a letter of complaint written by Mr Turner and copied to the Care Quality Commission. He appears to have been aware of the tension between Dr Jenkins and the prison officers and the main text of his complaint is that he was not offered the level of privacy and dignity which he would have received if he had been any other member of the public. He also complains that the site at which intravenous cannula which was inserted in his left antecubital fossa became inflamed and he required 7 days of antibiotics and dressings. He says Dr Jenkins appeared flustered and cross when inserting the cannula and as a result failed to take suitable antiseptic precautions or use a requisite level of skill.

### Expert opinion

The investigations and management plan undertaken by Dr Jenkins seem to have been entirely appropriate. She does however concede that the argument between her and the prison officers was difficult and she was very upset by it. Mr Turner was clearly aware of the differences of opinion voiced by both parties.

Prisoners have a right to expect a level of care commensurate with that afforded to all other patients in the NHS and that this includes a right to privacy, dignity and confidentiality. However, clearly at times there may be additional concerns about maintenance of security and the safety of healthcare professionals and these have to be taken into account. Dr Jenkins should have taken advice from a more senior colleague rather than get drawn into an open argument in front of the patient. A calmer discussion may have revealed a genuine reason for anxiety on the part of the prison officers that

*Avoiding Errors in Adult Medicine*, First Edition. Ian P. Reckless, D. John M. Reynolds, Sally Newman, Joseph E. Raine, Kate Williams and Jonathan Bonser.
© 2013 John Wiley & Sons, Ltd. Published 2013 by John Wiley & Sons, Ltd.

Dr Jenkins might not have been safe in the room on her own with Mr Turner. It is a concern however that Dr Jenkins is unable to participate meaningfully in any risk assessment given that she has been given no information as to why Mr Turner is in prison (nor is she entitled to any).

The presence of handcuffs made it impossible for Dr Jenkins to insert the cannula in a vein in the hand or wrist. It is important to be alert to the effects that being under pressure or being upset may have on the performance of routine tasks. It took Dr Jenkins several attempts to insert the line and she admits she couldn't wait to get out of the room.

## ⚠️ Legal comment

A prisoner or person in policy custody has the same right to confidentiality and to give or withhold consent as any other patient. Healthcare professionals should insist on making a full and proper clinical assessment. Some concessions for a prisoner/patient in custody may be proper, such as accelerating the patient to the department being mindful of the balance of risk and benefit to the safety of staff and others in the Emergency Department. It is important that healthcare professionals' integrity is not compromised. The fact that someone is a detained prisoner does not affect his right to be treated nor his right to consent or refuse to treatment nor his right to confidentiality.

It is proper to communicate details to his prison warders only if the patient consents. Dr Jenkins should have insisted on full access to the patient in order to permit her to make as full an assessment as any other patient. If a patient requires admission or any other treatment it must be offered irrespective of other considerations. If this is obstructed, it must be witnessed, documented and, if necessary, reported.

In this circumstance, taking a proper history in the presence of the prison warders was an infringement of the prisoner's human rights and impacted upon his dignity. If Dr Jenkins was finding it difficult to make a full assessment she should have recorded that the patient had not been properly assessed. It is important for Dr Jenkins to have discharged her duty of care to the patient. It would have been appropriate to insist that

the prison warders organize themselves so that proper conditions for the consultation existed even in the Emergency Department. It is essential to insist politely that a proper assessment must be made if the patient will allow it. If the patient refuses, this must be documented and senior help obtained from a Consultant.

NHS organizations have a duty to promote equality and social inclusion.

The duty to respect the individual's privacy to the greatest extent possible is not only a professional obligation but also a requirement of the Human Rights Act 1998. Any infringement of that right must be legitimate and proportionate. The Trust as a public authority has a duty to comply with the Human Rights Act 1998 that guarantees individuals under Article 8 the right to a private life.

The need to preserve the patient's privacy and dignity during examination or treatment must be balanced against the risk of danger to the healthcare professional. Consideration also should be had for the safety of Dr Jenkins in terms of chaperone or necessary security precautions depending on the security status of the prisoner. Some detainees have a history of violence or may become violent. In some cases the prison warder may advise the doctor to exercise caution in which case the normal practice would be to examine the prisoner with protection. Ideally the prison warder should be out of immediate earshot, although this depends on the circumstances.

In this case, the failure to obtain a proper medical history and to properly examine has resulted in pain and suffering for seven days. The prisoner therefore has a case in civil law for compensation for the Trust's breach of its duty of care to him.

### ⚠️ Key learning points

**General points**
- Keep calm in all clinical interactions and step away from the situation where necessary.
- Do not have arguments in front of patients.
- If you are upset defer practical procedures where possible.
- Seek advice from senior colleagues when you are in a situation you have not faced before.

# Case 25  Own worst enemy

The duty consultant chemical pathologist contacts the medical SHO on-call at 19.40 in the evening to inform him of an abnormal serum potassium (1.8 mmol/L) taken from an outpatient. The laboratory has been unable to contact the referrer (a GP) and asks the SHO to contact the patient and manage the situation. The clinical details given with the request state 'bulimia nervosa'. The SHO attempts to contact the patient, 21-year-old Ms Barnes, and speaks to her mother on the telephone. Ms Barnes refuses to talk to the SHO.

### Should the SHO speak to Ms Barnes's mother?

The SHO explains the situation to Ms Barnes's mother and she agrees to accompany Ms Barnes to the hospital.

In taking her history, the SHO discovers that Ms Barnes has had an eating disorder since the age of 15. She attended the hospital three weeks ago following a first episode of self-harm (cutting), having split up with her boyfriend. She has been vomiting (self-induced) since discharge from hospital. There is no history of laxative use. Ms Barnes complains of intermittent muscle cramps, particularly affecting the calves. On examination, Ms Barnes's body mass index is in the range of 16-18 kg/m$^2$. She has some lanugo hair on the cheeks and bilateral parotid swelling. She has been managed by her GP, Dr Green, and has blood tests performed fortnightly. She is withdrawn and avoids eye contact.

Repeat blood tests confirm profound hypokalaemia and Ms Barnes agrees to intravenous fluid administration but refuses oral potassium supplements. After 3 litres over 10 hours, Ms Barnes's serum potassium is measured at 3.4 mmol.

### What would you do now?

Ms Barnes suddenly becomes agitated and insists that she be allowed to go home. She says that she is fed up with people looking at her as if she was a circus animal. Ms Barnes's mother is tearful but seems resigned to Ms Barnes's outburst. She says that she will remain in the house with Ms Barnes during the afternoon and overnight.

### How would you decide whether Ms Barnes should be allowed to go home?

Ms Barnes appears to be orientated in time, place and person. The SHO allows her to go home and advises her to seek assistance from her GP the next day.

Three days later, the SHO comes into work and discover that Ms Barnes had thrown herself from a multi-storey car park the previous night. She has transected her spinal cord at C3 and is quadriplegic.

Six months later, Ms Barnes's mother takes legal action against the hospital claiming that the suicide attempt and resulting injuries could have been prevented had a formal risk assessment been undertaken.

### Expert opinion

Ms Barnes presented with an acute medical problem which was corrected appropriately. The SHO recognized that the discharge was risky but ensured that she would be accompanied and advised her to seek further help from her GP. The SHO felt that Ms Barnes was an adult who had been orientated and was communicating coherently. She had not expressed any suicidal ideation and the primary issue, bulimia, appeared to be chronic.

The SHO acted reasonably in the circumstances and the absence of a formal mental health and competency assessment is acceptable.

### Legal comment

There is an assumption that a patient of 21 years of age has capacity. One of the five core principles of the

*Avoiding Errors in Adult Medicine*, First Edition. Ian P. Reckless, D. John M. Reynolds, Sally Newman, Joseph E. Raine, Kate Williams and Jonathan Bonser.
© 2013 John Wiley & Sons, Ltd. Published 2013 by John Wiley & Sons, Ltd.

Mental Capacity Act (MCA) 2005 is that a person is assumed to have capacity unless it is established otherwise. The consent of the patient is required before personal information can be shared with a third party. If this patient had impaired capacity due to the abnormal serum potassium, then the doctor could take steps in her best interests so that she is brought to hospital quickly.

The conversation with Ms Barnes's mother would have to be carefully worded so that the urgent need for Ms Barnes to obtain emergency treatment was imparted without disclosing unnecessary confidential healthcare information.

The SHO would have had to have overriding evidence of a psychological condition requiring sectioning under the Mental Health Act 1983 in order to prevent Ms Barnes from taking her own discharge. It would have been important to elicit her past medical history and any desire to self-harm. To prevent Ms Barnes from taking her own discharge, the SHO would have to have evidence of a psychological condition which justified her being sectioned under the Mental Health Act.

In the absence of a documented assessment of the patient's capacity at the time of the decision to self-discharge, this case will be difficult to defend.

When where restraint needs to be used, staff will be protected from liability if certain conditions are met. These conditions are set out in Sections 5 and 6 of the MCA. They must reasonably believe that the patient lacks capacity to consent to the act in question, that the act needs to be done in the patient's best interests and that restraint is necessary to protect the person from harm. The restraint used must be a proportionate or reasonable response to the likelihood of the person suffering harm and to the seriousness of the potential harm.

## ⚠ Key learning points

### Specific to the case
- The mental state of all patients should be considered and when the presentation involves serious and sustained self-harm, a psychiatric opinion should be sought.
- Patients who are thought to pose a significant suicide risk can be detained until a formal assessment can be undertaken.

### General points
- Personal information in relation to a person with capacity cannot be shared with third parties (including relatives) without the implicit or explicit consent of that person.
- The Mental Capacity Act 2005 has become the vehicle for the temporary restraint of patients pending formal assessment (as opposed to Common law).

# Section 6: Miscellaneous

# Case 26  All eggs in one basket

Jade Nelson is a 34-year-old woman who self-presents in the emergency department because over the last two days she has experienced dull chest discomfort and feels out of breath when going upstairs, both of which are new symptoms for her. She is normally in reasonable health and with no significant previous medical history and no family history of note. She is overweight and smokes 20 cigarettes a day and her only regular medication is the combined oral contraceptive pill that she has taken for the last two years.

## What diagnoses are in your mind?

Mrs Nelson is seen by a CT1 in emergency medicine, Dr Fentiman, who finds her to be a little anxious, but he elicits no abnormalities on physical examination apart from a resting pulse rate of 90 and an oxygen saturation of 95%. The electrocardiogram confirms a sinus tachycardia and Mrs Nelson's chest X-ray is normal. The junior doctor requests a full blood count, basic biochemistry, and a D-dimer to help decide if she needs further imaging to rule out a pulmonary embolus. He calculates her pre-test probability for pulmonary embolism to be low using the Wells criteria.

Just after the blood samples have been sent, the hospital laboratory computer system fails with the effect that no blood results are available online. The problem persists for some hours and the delay in obtaining results to investigations slows the flow of patients through the Emergency Department, making a busy day more fraught for staff and patients alike.

## What should Dr Fentiman do?

After three hours, the laboratory phones through the results of Mrs Nelson's investigations and these are written down by a nurse who happens to be by the phone but who does not know Mrs Nelson. Dr Fentiman reviews the results and sees that the D-dimer is 398 and he concludes that Mrs Nelson is very low risk for having had a pulmonary embolism and requires no further investigation. By this time, some five hours after arrival in hospital, Mrs Nelson is feeling slightly better yet very frustrated. She is sent home with a putative diagnosis of a 'viral chest infection'.

The next day Dr Fentiman is again on duty and is called to attend to a patient in the resuscitation room who has suffered an out-of-hospital cardiac arrest. The resuscitation attempts fail and Dr Fentiman is distressed to find that the patient is Mrs Nelson who he sent home the day before.

A review of the previous day's investigations (now available online again) show the D-dimer was in fact 3980, not 398 as recorded following the telephone conversation. A coroner's post mortem examination later confirms that Mrs Nelson died following massive pulmonary embolism.

## Expert opinion

This case highlights a number of problem areas:

Dr Fentiman appears not to have considered what the mechanism of increased breathlessness and chest discomfort might have been in this young woman. There was no evidence in the notes of a logical differential diagnosis or a clear management plan. He used the Wells score to calculate a low pre-test probability of pulmonary embolism (prevalence <4%) but arguably without a clear alternative and more likely diagnosis for Mrs Nelson's symptoms he should have scored her at moderate risk (i.e. 21% prevalence).

The test result was communicated incorrectly – it is not clear whether the laboratory technician made an error or if the nurse who took the telephone call simply recorded the result incorrectly. Errors of this nature are worryingly common and in one study 3.5% of laboratory data communicated over the telephone were recorded incorrectly. The use of read-back to confirm

---

*Avoiding Errors in Adult Medicine*, First Edition. Ian P. Reckless, D. John M. Reynolds, Sally Newman, Joseph E. Raine, Kate Williams and Jonathan Bonser.
© 2013 John Wiley & Sons, Ltd. Published 2013 by John Wiley & Sons, Ltd.

that the information had been properly and accurately received abolished all of these errors.

The failure of the hospital results server during a busy time caused delay in processing patients and increased the pressure on staff. Delay also may have made patients more frustrated and could have made Mrs Nelson more likely to play down her problems and agree to go home. When systems do fail and staff have to revert to paper-based results and telephone communication it is all the more important that particular care is taken to ensure that results are correctly passed on.

When under pressure to process patients in a busy environment with the added strain of a system failure, it is easy to see how Mrs Nelson's symptoms and signs might be explained away. She is anxious and so the heart rate of 90 is dismissed, she is a smoker and the oxygen saturations of 95% were similarly ignored. It is always important to ask: 'what has changed to cause this otherwise well woman to attend the emergency department today'? In the absence of any infective symptoms, how likely is this presentation to be caused by a viral infection? How do viruses make you breathless (pneumonitis or unmasking of obstructive airways disease)?

## ⚠ Legal comment

A Trust-wide failure of laboratory results systems would trigger the Serious Incident Requiring Investigation (SIRI) process, given the number of patients whose safety could be adversely affected.

The coroner seeking the factual cause of death would need to consider the systems failures that entailed no test results for a number of hours, and jeopardizing patient safety. The coroner may consider a Rule 43 letter about not only the failure of the results system but also the poor practice that resulted in an incorrect test result being written down. It would help to reassure the coroner that a recurrence is unlikely if a completed clinical risk action plan/root cause analysis from the SIRI was provided to him, along with evidence of improved systems and back up contingencies to improve patient safety.

Simple changes in individual practice (for example, read-back) would reduce the danger of flawed clinical decision-making, improve patient safety and reduce litigation risk. The quality of documentation is crucial to the Trust's ability to defend itself against litigation.

As it is, since there is a three-year limitation period from the date of death, following the coroner's inquest, there could then be a civil action which would not be defensible.

Whilst it is important for the Trust to identify root causes and learning, it is equally important to ensure that support is offered to Dr Fentiman following the shock of recognizing Mrs Nelson during resuscitation. Effective risk management places an emphasis on openness rather than blame.

### ⚠ Key learning points

**General points**

- When a clinical area is busy and/or systems are under pressure, clinicians need to devote extra care to clinical decision making.
- Standardized operating protocols (SOP) can be useful in ensuring that rules are applied within complex and error-prone processes.

## References and further reading

Barenfanger J, Sautter RL, Lang DL, *et al.* (2004) Improving patient safety by repeating (Read-back) telephone reports of critical information. *Am J Clin Pathol* **121**: 801–3.

Reynard J, Reynolds J, Stevenson P (2009) *Practical Patient Safety.* Oxford University Press.

Wells PS, Anderson DR, Rodger M, *et al.* (2000) Derivation of a simple clinical model to categorize patients with a probability of pulmonary embolism: increasing the model's utility with the SimpliRED D-dimer. *Thromb Haemost* **83**: 416–20.

# Case 27  A major mix-up

Mr Johnson is a 68-year-old man who has type 2 diabetes and mild COPD. He becomes unwell at home with a fever and pleuritic chest pain but delays seeking medical help. By the time his GP is asked to see him, Mr Johnson is hypotensive with septic shock and an emergency admission to hospital is arranged.

## What treatments should be instituted upon Mr Johnson's arrival at hospital?

The core medical trainee who first sees Mr Johnson, Dr Hewitt, appreciates the gravity of the situation and immediately gives intravenous ceftriaxone, oxygen and intravenous saline and commences an insulin sliding scale. He also prescribes subcutaneous low molecular weight heparin for venous thromboprophylaxis. A chest X-ray shows widespread consolidation in the left lung field. Mr Johnson is significantly hypoxic with oxygen saturations of 82% despite 28% oxygen. Blood gases show he is acidotic with a pH of 6.99 and a lactate of 7 mmol/L. With aggressive fluid resuscitation, Mr Johnson's blood pressure increases and over the next hour or so he begins to improve.

On the post take ward round, the Consultant decides to administer intravenous sodium bicarbonate because Mr Johnson still has 'acidotic breathing' although his condition is now more stable and he is producing a good urine output and appears to be less confused.

## Do you agree with this decision?

Two hours later Mr Johnson suddenly becomes more unwell and rapidly loses consciousness. A cardiac arrest call is put out and on arrival the team find Mr Johnson to be asystolic. Despite a prolonged attempt to resuscitate him, Mr Johnson dies. As the arrest team are writing up the details of their treatment, the anaesthetic registrar asks 'Why he was he receiving iv lidocaine?' The nurse who had been looking after Mr Johnson denied he was, but on inspection it is clear that the pre-prepared and packaged giving set does indeed contain lidocaine and not bicarbonate as intended and prescribed clearly on the drug chart.

## Who should be informed of this death?

The case is reported to the coroner who refers it to the police. The police interview the nurse and ask him if he checked the infusion before connecting it up. The nurse says 'I couldn't have done' and at this stage he is cautioned by the police and informed he may be charged with manslaughter (although after a year, a decision is made not to pursue charges).

It later transpires that the nurse was working single handed in a very busy bay with three particularly sick patients. He did not feel he could ask for help to check the infusion when he set it up because his colleagues were similarly busy. He remembered seeing a box containing pre-packaged bicarbonate on the ward and went and picked one out to give to Mr Johnson. In fact the box did contain pre-packaged infusion bags of bicarbonate but somehow a single bag of lidocaine had been mixed in with the bicarbonate bags during a recent ward stock-taking exercise. Superficially the pre-packaged bags all look the same and the most prominent label is not the drug contained within them but rather the company trade name (in this case, Polyfusor®). The confusion was understandable but the checking had been too cursory to detect the similarity and avoid the problem.

Following on from this incident, the Health and Safety Executive undertook an investigation of the working environment. A number of factors were identified including the adequacy of lighting in the cupboard, the organization of supplies and the hours worked by the staff nurse concerned.

*Avoiding Errors in Adult Medicine*, First Edition. Ian P. Reckless, D. John M. Reynolds, Sally Newman, Joseph E. Raine, Kate Williams and Jonathan Bonser.
© 2013 John Wiley & Sons, Ltd. Published 2013 by John Wiley & Sons, Ltd.

## ⚙ Expert opinion

The initial management of Mr Johnson by the core medical trainee was appropriate and timely. The decision taken on the post-take ward round to prescribe bicarbonate was subsequently questioned as no further blood gas analysis had been undertaken and Mr Johnson was clearly improving. Bicarbonate is not without risk and may not have been required if the acidosis had significantly improved. The prescription for bicarbonate was clearly and correctly written and the nurse was asked in person to commence the infusion.

The use of pre-packaged infusions is an important way of avoiding errors that might otherwise occur in calculating and preparing or diluting an infusion. However the first error in this case was that a lidocaine bag had become mixed in with the bags of bicarbonate during a ward stock take. In fact some years earlier a similar episode had occurred and as a result of that all pre-packaged infusions of lidocaine had been removed from general wards and non-resuscitation areas. Unfortunately Mr Johnson was on the medical assessment unit where lidocaine was held as stock and there was a lack of awareness of the potential for confusion. It is a recurring theme that all too often products which superficially look alike are stored together.

This fatal drug administration error occurred because of a combination of system errors, a catalyst event and then simple human error. The system errors included inadequate staffing, leading to a stressful environment. The nurse was inexperienced and being asked to cover too many sick patients at once. The drug packaging was confusing and storage facilities were poor. The catalyst event was that unusually a stock take had occurred on the ward that day and all of the Polyfusor® bags placed in a single box. The human error was the failure to check adequately even though he did recall looking at the bag – in haste and presumably he saw what he wanted to see. Once the infusion bag had been set up and connected it is highly unlikely that the error was going to be picked up and the catastrophic outcome had been set in motion.

## ⚖ Legal comment

This adverse incident illustrates how one set of events can result in a number of appropriate investigations by different agencies. The unexpected death of the patient was reported to the coroner. Since one of the root causes of the patient's death was the action of the individual nurse in selecting the incorrect drug, the coroner appropriately informed the police. It is rare for healthcare professionals to be investigated for a criminal offence arising from patient deaths associated with clinical practice. As we have seen in other case studies, the more usual route for legal investigation and remedy of patient harm is through the civil system. Conviction for a criminal offence requires proof beyond reasonable doubt that the person charged has carried out an unlawful act (*actus reus*) and had the state of mind (or intention) to carry out the act (*mens rea*). Both elements must be present for a successful criminal prosecution.

The police and Crown Prosecution Service (CPS) considered a charge of manslaughter by gross negligence against the nurse. The charges of murder and manslaughter are distinguished by the state of mind of the defendant. In this case study, the actions of the nurse were part of the cause of the patient's death; but the nurse did not have any intention to kill or cause serious injury to the patient. The definition of manslaughter by gross negligence requires the existence of a duty of care; breach of that duty; death occurring as a consequence of the breach of duty and a reckless disregard for the safety of others justifying a criminal conviction. In the context of this case study, the CPS needed to assess if a jury would consider the nurse had appreciated the risk and intended to avoid it, but displayed such a high degree of negligence in the attempted avoidance as to justify conviction for inattention/failure to advert a serious risk in respect of an obvious matter.

It is important to remember to retain the evidence (for example, the Polyfusor® bag) in any adverse incident in case items are required as evidence by the coroner or the police.

## ⚠ Key learning points

### General points

• Medical error may occur when a weak point in an apparently straightforward process converges with the weak point in another related process (for example, the automated checking of patient identity in radiology fails at the same time as a shift handover for porters – and two patients are returned to the wrong ward area) – James Reason's Swiss Cheese Model.
• Manslaughter convictions are rare in healthcare.

## Reference

Reason J (1990) *Human Error*. Cambridge University Press.

# Case 28 Under the radar

Victor M'shangwe is a 36-year-old Zimbabwean living in the United Kingdom. Mr M'shangwe is usually fit and well. Over the last 7–10 days, he has become progressively more short of breath. He has a cough productive of green phlegm and has had drenching sweats. In the last 24 hours he has developed severe pleuritic pain and attends the Emergency Department where he is seen by Dr Williams, a core trainee in Acute Care Common Stem (ACCS).

## What should be the key elements of Dr Williams' management plan?

Dr Williams takes a history from Mr M'shangwe and examines him. He has not travelled outside the UK in the last two years. She identifies bronchial breath sounds above a small pleural effusion at the right base. Mr M'shangwe has a heart rate of 90 and a systolic blood pressure of 105 mmHg. Oxygen saturations are 96% on room air and the respiratory rate is 18 min$^{-1}$. His temperature is 38 °C. Dr Williams draws routine bloods, blood cultures and, considering a diagnosis of community acquired lobar pneumonia to be likely, obtains verbal consent for an HIV test. She requests a chest X-ray and prescribes a nonsteroidal anti-inflammatory drug.

## Would you have acted differently?

Blood tests show a neutrophilia and a C-reactive protein (CRP) of 105. Tests of liver and renal function are within normal limits. The chest radiograph confirms consolidation in the right lower lobe and a small pleural effusion. Dr Williams explains to Mr M'shangwe that he has a lobar pneumonia. She prescribes a course of oral amoxicillin in line with local guidelines and tells Mr M'shangwe to take regular paracetamol and drink plenty of fluid in the days ahead. She explains to Mr M'shangwe that if he feels worse rather than better, he ought to return for a further assessment as an empyema may develop. She asks him to go to his GP later in the week for the results of the HIV test and blood cultures. She explains that Mr M'shangwe will be contacted by the hospital if blood cultures grow bacteria which are not responsive to amoxicillin.

At this point, Mr M'shangwe tells Dr Williams that he does not have a GP and that he is in the country illegally, an earlier application for asylum having been refused. Dr Williams agrees to contact Mr M'shangwe through a friend's mobile telephone to provide the HIV results later in the week.

Two days later, Dr Williams looks up Mr M'shangwe's HIV result and finds it to be positive. Before calling the patient, she asks her consultant, Dr Gupta, how she should direct Mr M'shangwe in order that he can access appropriate treatment. Dr Gupta consults with colleagues in the Trust's GUM department and is surprised to find that the Trust is not able to provide treatment in these circumstances. A Trust policy states that long-term HIV treatment does not constitute emergency treatment and that patients can only be offered treatment where they have full eligibility to NHS care. Mr M'shangwe would be able to purchase the appropriate medications but he cannot receive them on the NHS.

Dr Williams telephones Mr M'shangwe and explains both the HIV result and the situation regarding treatment to him. She is apologetic but explains that her hands are tied. She offers advice in relation to unprotected sexual intercourse. Mr M'shangwe does not feel that he has the resources to access treatment privately.

## What do you think of the trust's stance? Is the trust acting within the law?

A fortnight later, the Trust receives a letter from a local human rights advocacy group sent on behalf of

*Avoiding Errors in Adult Medicine*, First Edition. Ian P. Reckless, D. John M. Reynolds, Sally Newman, Joseph E. Raine, Kate Williams and Jonathan Bonser.
© 2013 John Wiley & Sons, Ltd. Published 2013 by John Wiley & Sons, Ltd.

Mr M'shangwe. The letter, copied to the local commissioning group, the local MP and the Secretary of State for Health, challenges the Trust's position on the prescription of anti-retrovirals and points out that Mr M'shangwe would not have access to treatment if he were to return to Zimbabwe and also that his HIV constitutes a potential public health threat whilst untreated in the UK.

## Expert opinion

The medical aspects here are straightforward. Dr William's treatment was appropriate. It was reasonable to have discharged Mr M'shangwe for outpatient treatment given his presentation and his low CURB-65 risk score. Lack of eligibility to NHS care is often a challenging issue to deal with from an ethical perspective, perhaps because NHS clinicians are so used to the idea of treatment free at the point of need. The legal aspect is relatively clear. Individuals can only receive NHS treatment if they are entitled to it – broadly this includes citizens of the European Union (with some caveats applying to accession countries) and those with formal refugee or asylum status. Individuals who do not have the right to remain in the country, or who are present informally 'under the radar' are generally not eligible for NHS treatment.

NHS Trusts may apply these rules rather more flexibly in Emergency Departments and, to an extent, sexual health clinics. In these environments, treatment is generally provided: questions of eligibility and if relevant, efforts to recoup costs through charging, are usually deferred. In outpatients, or following admission (elective or emergency), patients without entitlement should be charged for the treatment they receive. At present, there is no requirement for the NHS body to break confidentiality and inform other authorities of the presence of a patient in a hospital who does not have the right to remain. A doctor prescribing privately for a patient would not be compelled to take legal or immigration status into account.

Whilst a patient without legal right to be in the United Kingdom might be treated (perhaps against their will) for conditions such as multi-drug resistant TB, the public health argument has not been accepted in relation to HIV therapy. The patient has the ability to prevent transmission through appropriate precautions and sexual abstinence. Differential access to life saving treatments between country of origin and the United Kingdom has not, to date, been extensively supported in immigration Case Law.

## Legal comment

Emergency and life-saving treatment will always be given in ED free at the point of delivery to all patients. Where the patient is not a UK resident, then under reciprocal arrangements with, for example, European Union countries or through the patient's travel insurance, the Trust will seek reimbursement of costs of treatment. Under most travel insurance agreements, the Trust has a duty to care for the patient until fit to travel back to the country of origin.

The problems with charging for overseas visitors escalate if the patient requires ongoing chronic treatment. It is very important for the Trust to check the patient's residential status and eligibility for free treatment when he is being considered for continued admission in hospital or for ongoing chronic treatment, e.g. dialysis for renal failure.

Article 2 of the Human Rights Act 1998, the right to life, is usually only quoted when applicants for asylum have been diagnosed with a chronic condition, and the absence of medical treatment in their country of origin is raised as a human rights issue for the authorities considering deportation.

All Trusts have an overseas patient manager, who is available to meet with patients to ascertain ability to pay and residential status (which may exempt payment).

Until recently, patients without residential legal status have not been able to access free treatment for HIV in England, despite arguments based on cost effectiveness (reduced costs compared with the subsequent treatment of AIDS) and public health (reduced potential for onward transmission). Amendments to the Health and Social Care Bill 2011 as it passed through Parliament during the course of 2012 provide for free treatment for patients who have been in the UK for over six months (irrespective of legal status). This should lead to changes in the years ahead, bringing England in line with Scotland and Wales (where free treatment for HIV is provided to patients not ordinarily eligible for NHS care).

## Key learning points

### General points
• Patients who are neither citizens nor residents of the European Union are unlikely to be entitled to free NHS care

## Reference and further reading

BBC News (2012) Free HIV treatment on NHS for foreign nationals, 28 February 2012. http://www.bbc.co.uk/news/health-17187179 [last accessed 01 June 2012].

Lim WS, van der Eerden MM, Laing R, *et al.* (2003) Defining community acquired pneumonia severity on presentation to hospital: an international derivation and validation study. *Thorax* **58** (5): 377–82.

# Case 29 A cantankerous recluse

Mr Peacock is a 78-year-old reclusive man who has lived alone in a static caravan in rather precarious circumstances for many years. He drinks about 60 units of alcohol a week and is a heavy smoker. He is admitted to hospital somewhat reluctantly after a fall which he thinks occurred when he slipped climbing up the steps to his home. He is unable to mobilize because he feels generally too weak and he is in pain. When he is first assessed he is uncooperative and abusive to staff and refuses to get out of his bed. It is clear that he is unkempt and he has bilateral leg ulcers which have not been dressed adequately for some time but which he denies cause him pain. He has a probable fracture of his right arm and he appears to be in urinary retention.

### Are there any particular diagnoses that it would be important to consider?

After reassurance and some tea and food he agrees to be undressed, cleaned up and for some investigations to be done. X-rays show hyper-expanded lung fields, and a fracture of his right humerus. He has a raised white count and CRP and no other significant abnormalities. He agrees to analgesia (paracetamol and codeine), a sling for his arm, and to urinary catheterization. Just over a litre of urine is drained and dip testing shows leucocytes and nitrites so he is also given co-amoxiclav orally for five days.

The Consultant who sees him on the post-take ward round adds in intravenous B vitamins and some regular chlordiazepoxide to cover likely alcohol withdrawal. Mr Peacock remains suspicious of staff and refuses to be examined again and will not get out of bed. Overnight he becomes more aggressive and confused and falls again when he tries to get up. The next morning things have settled, but Mr Peacock remains mildly confused which is put down to his infection and alcohol withdrawal. The GP is contacted in order to get a fuller picture, but it is clear that Mr Peacock has kept away from the practice

for some years and has a reputation locally for being eccentric.

Over the weekend Mr Peacock seems to improve and he becomes less suspicious of people trying to help him and he no longer seems confused. The nursing notes record that he is constipated and the cover FY1 is asked to write up a laxative.

### Are you content with Mr Peacock's management to date?

On Monday the hospital is very busy and as a bed has become available in a nurse-led local community hospital, Mr Peacock is moved from the acute ward. A rushed handover note is written by a junior doctor who has not met Mr Peacock before.

A week later the nursing staff in the community hospital ask the GP to visit because they cannot persuade Mr Peacock to get out of bed or cooperate with any rehabilitation. The GP is worried that Mr Peacock cannot raise his legs from the bed, he remains constipated (despite stopping the codeine and having regular laxatives) and now has developed pressure sores on his heels. He is referred back to acute hospital and seen again on-take, 12 days after the initial fall at home. The admitting registrar is concerned that Mr Peacock has spinal cord compression and he arranges an MRI scan which shows severe lumbar spinal stenosis and cauda equina compression from an L4/5 disc protrusion. Surgical decompression is undertaken the next day but Mr Peacock's recovery is incomplete. Several months later he remains permanently catheterized, and is unable to stand unaided. He develops severe recurrent urinary sepsis with vancomycin resistant enterococci, and his pressure sores are very slow to resolve.

The GP writes a letter to the Chief Executive of the hospital saying he believes that the diagnosis was so delayed that the chances of recovery were compromised. He also complains about the pressure sores, the poor quality of the handover, the rushed circumstances of

*Avoiding Errors in Adult Medicine*, First Edition. Ian P. Reckless, D. John M. Reynolds, Sally Newman, Joseph E. Raine, Kate Williams and Jonathan Bonser.
© 2013 John Wiley & Sons, Ltd. Published 2013 by John Wiley & Sons, Ltd.

the transfer to the community hospital and the hospital acquired infection. The hospital responds by designating this as a serious incident requiring investigation (SIRI) and arranges an internal enquiry.

## 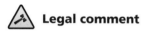 Expert opinion

The overriding sense one gets with the management of Mr Peacock is that no one appears to have taken his symptoms seriously because he was rude and difficult with staff. Attempts to undertake a functional assessment on admission were indeed thwarted by the confusion and lack of engagement but it is clear that no neurological examination was undertaken and inadequate thought given to the possibility that the retention, constipation and reluctance to mobilize might have had a more serious underlying cause. Any delay in resolving cord and cauda equina compression may contribute to suboptimal long-term recovery.

Mr Peacock's attitude to staff almost certainly made it more difficult to reach a diagnosis and also for nursing staff to undertake simple but essential monitoring of his pressure areas but both the medical and nursing notes fail to document adequate attempts to look beyond his behavioural difficulties and identify the underlying problem.

## Legal comment

The GP's letter of complaint will receive a formal letter of response from the Chief Executive under the Trust's Complaints Process. Since all aspects of Mr Peacock's care have also been subject to a SIRI investigation, the formal complaint response letter may enclose a copy of the final SIRI report as this will include a factual chronology of events and confirmation of the Trust's completed action plan.

The GP would not have any *locus standi* (i.e. no legal position) to initiate legal action on behalf of the patient against the Trust. Mr Peacock would need to instruct solicitors himself. A motivating factor for civil action would be the ongoing symptoms and care that Mr Peacock requires.

The assessment of liability would focus on the issue of causation. No neurological examination was undertaken and there was therefore a delay to definitive management. Expert evidence will be required to assist in determining whether, on balance of probability, earlier diagnosis might have permitted improved long-term recovery.

Mr Peacock's inpatient fall should have triggered the Trust's incident reporting process and retrospective root cause analysis. However, it is well known that only a minority of incidents are reported through formal systems which makes it difficult to know the true incidence of patient harm.

## Key learning points

### Specific to the case
• Where an appropriate examination is not feasible at a particular point in time, clinicians must ensure that reasonable attempts are made to complete the comprehensive assessment at another time, or a clear estimation of the risks and benefits of an alternative management strategy is articulated.

### General points
• Hospitals are increasingly busy and hectic places with ever more pressure to maintain patient flow. Patient safety must always be considered when making efforts to redesign processes and improve operational efficiency. The quality of handover is particularly important.

# Case 30  Keep an open mind

Mr Watkins is a 61-year-old man who brings himself up to the Emergency Department because he is unwell with vomiting and abdominal pain. The triage nurse finds him to be clammy, vomiting and in obvious distress. His blood pressure is 196/103, his heart rate 50 beats per minute, his temperature 34.4 °C and his respiratory rate 28 breaths per minute. Oxygen saturations are 98% on room air. The nurse asks the medical FY2, Dr Singleton to see Mr Watkins. Dr Singleton undertakes a prompt assessment, inserts an intravenous line and administers a litre of normal saline along with 8 mg morphine (titrated to pain) and 10 mg of metoclopramide. Dr Singleton thinks Mr Watkins probably has an acute gastroenteritis but also wonders about pancreatitis. He sends off blood for electrolytes, haematology, amylase and liver function tests before arranging chest and plain abdominal X-rays.

Half an hour later Mr Watkins is much more settled and his son arrives to see him. Shortly afterwards Dr Singleton hears the son shouting, 'come quickly, Dad can't breathe'.

## What possibilities should cross Dr Singleton's mind?

When Dr Singleton enters the cubicle, he finds Mr Watkins deeply cyanosed with oxygen saturations of 50%. He is making ineffectual respiratory efforts and Dr Singleton suggests to the attending nurse that airway obstruction seems likely. However, on careful examination he cannot identify any obstruction. Dr Singleton administers 400 mg of naloxone in case this is respiratory arrest caused by the morphine he gave earlier. He inserts an endotracheal tube (without any difficulty or resistance from the patient) and manually bags Mr Watkins whose saturations rapidly improve. Throughout all of this Mr Watkins's blood pressure and pulse have been maintained.

Gradually Mr Watkins begins to breathe spontaneously and he is extubated. A CT pulmonary angiogram is arranged urgently in case this was respiratory arrest caused by a pulmonary embolism, but no clot is seen on the scan. The radiologist also scans Mr Watkins's neck and comments that there is no evidence of any obstructing lesion around the airway. Over the next 24 hours Mr Watkins recovers fully from both his presenting complaint and from his respiratory arrest. Dr Singleton is perturbed by the turn of events, which he is struggling to explain, but rationalizes that maybe this was all caused by an unusual reaction to the intravenous morphine he had administered. He discusses it with his Consultant but no further action is taken.

## Should Dr Singleton have considered any other course of action?

Five weeks later another case arises in the Emergency Department where a patient becomes inexplicably hypoglycaemic and the consultant on duty writes in the notes 'it is difficult to explain the sequence of events'. He discusses the case with risk management and with his colleagues who all chip in with their recent experiences in the Emergency Department. It becomes clear that there have been ten unusual clinical events in the preceding three months and a very rapid internal investigation is triggered that day. It soon becomes apparent that deliberate harm cannot be ruled out and when on-call rotas are examined one individual stands out as having been present for all 10 cases. The police are involved and a nurse is arrested when arriving at work on the following Monday morning.

The nurse is subsequently charged and found guilty of 2 counts of murder and 16 counts of grievous bodily harm. Forensic tests show that the nurse had variously and inappropriately administered vecuronium, midazolam and insulin to patients in the emergency department. Mr Watkins was almost certainly

*Avoiding Errors in Adult Medicine*, First Edition. Ian P. Reckless, D. John M. Reynolds, Sally Newman, Joseph E. Raine, Kate Williams and Jonathan Bonser.
© 2013 John Wiley & Sons, Ltd. Published 2013 by John Wiley & Sons, Ltd.

administered vecuronium and suffered 'dry drowning'. He subsequently recalled the nurse injecting something into the intravenous line in his arm and then almost immediately being unable to breathe. He remained conscious but unable to communicate throughout the emergency activity that then ensued. Fortunately he survived and suffered no long-term physical harm.

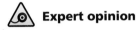

## Expert opinion

As Sherlock Holmes says in *The Sign of Four*, 'when you have eliminated the impossible, whatever remains, *however improbable*, must be the truth'. In a healthcare context it is all too easy to rationalize the seemingly inexplicable and one probably will feel that it is always more likely that a genuine medical complication is presenting in an unusual way than that a colleague may be deliberately setting out to cause harm. However, even though deliberate harm of this nature is fortunately rare, unexplained complications do arise much more frequently from drug dispensing or administration errors and you should always be prepared to consider that somewhere along the line an error might have occurred. Be particularly vigilant when hypoglycaemia arises in a patient who has previously been stable and who is not receiving insulin or hypoglycaemic agents.

Whenever you propose a diagnosis or explanation ensure the facts fit the mechanism you propose. Be logical and analytical – it is why you spent years learning basic anatomy, physiology, biochemistry, pharmacology and pathology.

## Legal comment

When senior clinical staff are presented with sufficient evidence for reasonable grounds to suspect that deliberate harm has occurred, contact should be made with the local police Criminal Investigation Department (CID). The Trust will have established relationships with the local police both through both the Trust legal team and Trust security department. There will often be a hospital police liaison officer and there is an overarching memorandum of understanding between the NHS and the police. If a decision is taken out of hours, then the duty executive would be the person from the Trust to contact the police. Conviction for a criminal offence requires proof beyond reasonable doubt that the person charged has carried out an unlawful act (*actus reus*) and in doing so had the necessary state of mind (*mens rea*).

In addition under PACE (Police and Criminal Evidence) codes of practice, all citizens have a duty to help police officers to prevent crime and to discover offenders. This is a civic rather than a legal duty. When first notified, the police will advise on the preservation of evidence. Any subsequent clinical risk investigation must not interfere with the initial police enquiry by either contaminating evidence or interfering with potential witnesses before a criminal prosecution. Consent will be required from all patients to whose care the police suspect the healthcare professional contributed.

Organizational learning for the Trust only takes place after the police investigation and prosecution. In the meantime, the Trust's Human Resources Department would advise on suspension under the Trust's Conduct/Disciplinary Action Procedure. The paramount duty is to protect other patients from harm whilst investigations are on-going. The Trust's clinical risk teams are available to discuss concerns on an anonymous basis. An initial telephone call to raise the possibility that an individual may be causing deliberate harm to patients would be rapidly escalated. An initial meeting would be set up quickly to decide the best course of action for the Trust, including making contact with the appropriate external agencies.

## Key learning points

### General points
- Malevolent and criminal behaviour on the part of healthcare professionals is rare but it can and does occur.

### Further reading

The Shipman Inquiry (2005) http://www.shipman-inquiry.org.uk [last accessed 01 June 2012].

# Case 31  Healthcare acquired infection?

Mrs Sanderson is a 58-year-old lady with a long history of alcohol dependency. She presents to the medical take with a vague history of lethargy, malaise and nonspecific abdominal pain coming on over the last month or so. Her GP's letter states that the main trigger for admission is a heightened level of concern amongst Mrs Sanderson's family, most notably her daughter Jane who worries that Mrs Sanderson's already chaotic lifestyle is now at breaking point. Dr Jennings, an ST2 in core medicine, clerks Mrs Sanderson upon her arrival in hospital.

Mrs Sanderson appears lethargic and malnourished but does not display any focal neurology. She admits to drinking approximately 200 units of alcohol per week, typically as wine. She last drank 14 hours previously. She complains of generalized abdominal tenderness but on examination, the abdomen is soft and nontender with normal bowel sounds. Mrs Sanderson is sweaty and a little tremulous. She is unsteady on her feet. Observations show that Mrs Sanderson is apyrexial with a blood pressure of 115/56 and a regular pulse of 92. The chest is clear and a small area of erythema is noted over Mrs Sanderson's lower thoracic spine although the skin does not appear to be broken. The admitting nurse has undertaken bedside urinalysis which shows the presence of leucocytes and nitrites.

## What is the differential diagnosis, what investigations would you arrange and what treatment would you institute?

Dr Jennings sends routine blood tests including inflammatory markers and orders a chest radiograph. The urine specimen is sent to the laboratory for microscopy, culture and sensitivities. Whilst waiting for the blood results, Dr Jennings prescribes intravenous Pabrinex® and benzodiazepines in view of the significant alcohol history and apparent malnutrition. She elects not to commence antibiotics in the absence of cardiovascular compromise or clear urinary symptoms.

Blood tests show elevated inflammatory markers (ALP and CRP) with a modest elevation in the white cell count with a neutrophilia. Tests of hepatic synthetic function are normal. In addition to the neutrophilia, the full blood count demonstrates a low platelet count and a normocytic anaemia (7.6 g/dl). Mrs Sanderson's last recorded haemoglobin had been 10.3 g/dl (with a macrocytosis).

## What further tests would you consider in relation to the anaemia?

Dr Jennings requests a blood film and haematinics. The next day, the urine specimen is reported as showing mixed growth and haematinics show reduced serum iron, increased ferritin and elevated total iron binding capacity. The consultant considers these results to be consistent with iron deficiency and orders an inpatient OGD (in view of the alcohol excess) to be followed by a CT colon examination. On day 2, Mrs Sanderson is less tremulous and gives a more coherent history. She continues to describe a generalized abdominal discomfort but is able to eat, drink and mobilize.

An OGD shows mild gastritis without varices. The CT colon examination is undertaken as an inpatient and it demonstrates a normal bowel but widespread disc destruction and established vertebral body osteomyelitis throughout the thoracic and upper lumbar spine. Blood cultures are taken which confirm the presence of an MRSA bacteraemia.

## What should be done now?

Mrs Sanderson is commenced on intravenous vancomycin and has an echocardiogram performed which is

*Avoiding Errors in Adult Medicine*, First Edition. Ian P. Reckless, D. John M. Reynolds, Sally Newman, Joseph E. Raine, Kate Williams and Jonathan Bonser.
© 2013 John Wiley & Sons, Ltd. Published 2013 by John Wiley & Sons, Ltd.

normal. The Trust triggers the Serious Incident Requiring Investigation (SIRI) process in accordance with local and national guidelines. The bacteraemia is reported to the Department of Health through the Health Protection Agency.

A root cause analysis is undertaken locally which reveals a 24 hour admission to hospital four months prior to this presentation when Mrs Sanderson had fainted whilst shopping. Records show that she had been given two litres of intravenous saline whilst observed in the Clinical Decision Unit. No documentation was found in relation to the insertion or care of an intravenous cannula.

In respect of the current admission, minor procedural irregularities are noted in relation to a lack of cutaneous skin screening on admission in line with Trust policy. It is felt that the MRSA bacteraemia was probably acquired many weeks prior to admission, most likely related to the poor state of Mrs Sanderson's skin and the pressure damage noted over the lower thoracic spine. However, the investigation team were unable to rule out a connection with the cannula inserted in the Emergency Department when she had been admitted after the faint.

## ⚠ Expert opinion

Although staphylococcal bacteraemia usually has an aggressive course and is associated with a high mortality, it can on occasion present much more indolently as on this occasion. The diagnosis was made fortuitously on account of Mrs Sanderson's CT colon examination: this examination was only undertaken so quickly as she remained an inpatient for other reasons, and it could be argued that a conventional colonoscopy examination would in fact have been more appropriate.

The MRSA bacteraemia was investigated according to the formalized process put in place by the Strategic Health Authority as part of a national effort to reduce the burden of staphylococcal bacteraemia.

In this case, it may be that the hospital had nothing to do with the acquisition of the bacteraemia. The use of devices (intravenous cannulae, urinary catheters etc.) may well have been appropriate although there is a dearth of information on Mrs Sanderson's brief admission with the faint. At best, failure to deliver care in accordance with the Trust's own standards (MRSA screening on admission, poor documentation around cannula insertion) leaves an impression of suboptimal care.

## ⚖ Legal comment

As described in section one "negligence" is a breach of a duty of care. The doctors employed by the Trust will not be deemed to have acted negligently if they have acted in accordance with the opinion of a responsible body of medical practitioners, skilled and practised in that art.

In this case, whilst the root cause analysis has identified some aspects of the patient's care which were in contravention of the Trust's guidelines, even if staff had acted in accordance with the Trust's guidelines, the outcome may still have been the same. Moreover, the Trust's guidelines are only a guide to staff. Non-compliance is not necessarily evidence of suboptimal and negligent care. But if the Trust's guidelines are evidence-based or a reiteration of national guidelines or professional protocols, this lends weight to an expectation that a doctor should act a specific manner, and unless there is a good reason, a failure to do so is outside of the accepted responsible body of professional practice.

Solicitors acting for patients will often request copies of the Trust's guidelines or protocols as evidence of proper standards of care. The trend will continue as the National Institute for Health and Care Excellence makes further recommendations. Trust and national guidelines, however, while considered indicative of an accepted course of clinical practice, are not the benchmark for professional standards. Nevertheless, a clinical negligence claim pleaded on the basis that guidelines or protocols have been transgressed without good reason makes a strong case (Part 1, Section 1, Failure to follow protocols). But it should not be forgotten that before a patient is entitled to compensation, it must be proved that, on the balance of probability, the failure of the Trust staff to act in accordance with the guidelines was the direct cause of the patient's injury. In this case it seems likely that the MRSA was acquired weeks before hospital admission and so the Trust would have a causation defence.

NHS Trusts are required to register with the Care Quality Commission and comply with CQC standards. Some of these standards relate to infection control. Executive directors and operational managers are responsible for ensuring that staff know what is expected of them and for ensuring that the Trust complies. By means of a risk register, the Trust can monitor any difficulties in implementing guidelines. If there are problems, an action plan should be devised to overcome them.

The Corporate Manslaughter and Corporate Homicide Act 2007 introduced a new criminal offence for public authorities. A named executive director may be guilty if it is found that he or she was a controlling mind in an organisation whose decisions have beyond reasonable doubt caused a death.

The standard of proof both for this offence and for manslaughter by medical negligence is high, and so convictions are infrequent.

### ⚠ Key learning points

**Specific to the case**
- Staphylococcal bacteraemia can present in an indolent manner.

**General points**
- The Care Quality Commission's licensing regime provides a clear mechanism through which NHS organizations can be forced to cease operating.
- The Corporate Manslaugther and Corporate Homicide Act 2007 can render named executives criminally responsible for the shortcomings of NHS organizations.

# Case 32  Backing the wrong horse

Mr Moses, a 46-year-old primary school teacher of Afro-Caribbean origin, was referred to the medical take with right-sided ear ache, headache and general malaise on a background of a three week history of right facial weakness. The latter had been treated by Mr Moses's GP as probable Bell's palsy with steroids and aciclovir.

Mr Moses had a history of genital herpes two years prior. Travel history included a camping trip to the New Forest three months ago.

On examination, Mr Moses was found by the SHO to be drowsy but easily roused. His facial muscles appeared generally weak (lower motor neurone pattern) and he was unsteady on his feet. There was some neck stiffness and plantars were down-going.

## What would you advise?

In view of the bilateral facial palsy and the deteriorating conscious level, the Consultant considered meningo-encephalitis secondary to either herpes infection or Lyme disease to be the likely diagnosis. Broad spectrum antibiotics and aciclovir were given pending CT and a lumbar puncture.

Prior to lumbar puncture, serum calcium was found to be elevated at 3.03 and a chest X-ray demonstrated the presence of bilateral hilar enlargement. The working diagnosis was revised to neurosarcoidosis. Prednisolone was recommended and fluids were administered.

The next day, a subtle papular rash began to develop. Skin and conjunctival biopsies were arranged, along with serum ACE levels and an MRI scan of the parotids, in order to assist in the confirmation of a diagnosis of sarcoidosis. The patient was discharged to return to the outpatient clinic for review and results five days later.

## Any other possible diagnoses?

Mr Moses returned to hospital the day before his planned clinic appointment with insomnia, leg weakness and a metallic taste in the mouth. A number of small lymph nodes were identified on examination and a biopsy was arranged. Results from the previous admission were now available including serum ACE within the normal range and a skin biopsy consistent with fungal infection. Repeat bloods showed serum calcium of 3.56 and a white cell count elevated at 25 000. A blood film demonstrated the presence of circulating lymphoblasts.

A clinical haematology opinion was organized and a working diagnosis of HTLV-1 associated adult T-cell lymphoblastic lymphoma was made.

Mr Moses received urgent systemic chemotherapy with intra-thecal methotrexate. He subsequently relapsed and received several more courses of chemotherapy. No HLA-matched donor was available and Mr Moses died eight months after diagnosis.

## Expert opinion

It is possible that Mr Moses's diagnosis could have been made a number of days earlier had the link between hypercalcaemia in a patient of afro-Caribbean origin and T-cell lymphoblastic lymphoma been appreciated by the admitting team. This link is readily recognized within haematological circles but not amongst general physicians.

The admitting team, and the other specialties called upon to provide an opinion, were all rather blinkered in their quest to 'confirm sarcoid' rather than to approach the case from a more objective standpoint and constructively question that working diagnosis at every turn. It seems that the lymphadenopathy identified on readmission had developed very acutely along with the peripheral blood abnormalities. These two findings made the possibility of haematological malignancy obvious and it is difficult to avoid use of a 'retrospectoscope' once it is acquired. It is unclear whether a subtler degree of lymphadenopathy was present and should have been detected upon the initial presentation.

*Avoiding Errors in Adult Medicine*, First Edition. Ian P. Reckless, D. John M. Reynolds, Sally Newman, Joseph E. Raine, Kate Williams and Jonathan Bonser.
© 2013 John Wiley & Sons, Ltd. Published 2013 by John Wiley & Sons, Ltd.

In Mr Moses's case, the short delay in the diagnosis of a rare but devastating illness was of no consequence – appropriate measures had been put in place to manage the hypercalcaemia and appropriate follow up had been arranged to see through the result of the investigations that had been ordered.

## ⚠ Legal comment

When does making a clinical error equate to negligence? The recognition of the link between hypercalcaemia and T-cell lymphoma is recognized in the clinical sub-specialty of haematology. When assessing the duty of care of the general physician, for example, it is unlikely that a responsible body of medical opinion would have been aware of the link. As such, this failure to diagnose is unlikely to have been negligent. In this case even though there was an error in diagnosis, the causative link, between this admission and patient's death does not exist. On the balance of probability, the outcome would have been the same in any event. Any error was not the single direct cause of the patient's death.

## ⚠ Key learning points

### Specific to the case
- T cell lymphoma should be considered as a cause of hypercalcaemia in the Afro-Caribbean population.

### General points
- A finding of negligence requires a breach of the duty of care and a causation link.
- Whether or not a doctor acted reasonably will be judged against the actions of a responsible body of clinical peers.

# Case 33  A surprising turn of events

Mrs Whittaker is a 68-year-old lady who has been referred to the Acute Medical Unit (AMU) from the Emergency Department. Mrs Whittaker had been visiting her daughter Samantha, an inpatient on the gynaecology ward, when she had collapsed a couple of moments before the end of visiting hours. A staff nurse who witnessed the episode described how Mrs Whittaker had let out a loud scream before slumping gradually to the floor, her eyes closed, before exhibiting coarse rhythmical movements of the upper limbs, associated with grunting sounds. The episode had lasted for approximately five minutes. Following the episode, Mrs Whittaker appeared mute and was staring blankly forward but seemed physically stable and orientated. Samantha explained to the staff nurse that Mrs Whittaker had occasional fits and that she had been started on a medication by her GP following an appointment with a neurologist, Professor Raymont.

## What do you think is the likely diagnosis?

Dr Wallace, the Core Medical Trainee on duty, is not entirely sure what to make of Mrs Whittaker's presentation. The episode does not sound to be typical of epilepsy and there were no features to suggest a cardiac aetiology. Against this, Dr Wallace notes with interest the neurological review and commencement of medication. He elects to send some basic blood tests, undertake a urinary dipstick, and observe Mrs Whittaker overnight. Dr Wallace's Consultant reviews Mrs Whittaker at 21.30 that evening and agrees with the plan for overnight observation. Mrs Whittaker then states that she is sure she will be feeling better by morning. She is fully orientated although she says she has poor recollection of the episode.

The next morning, Dr Wallace reviews Mrs Whittaker first thing. The nurses report no problems overnight. Dr Wallace tells Mrs Whittaker that she can be discharged at which point she refuses point blank to go home. She states that her husband has dementia, that he spends the weekly household budget on prostitutes and escorts, and that every so often he hits and kicks her.

## What should Dr Wallace do?

Dr Wallace is considering what he ought to do next when the Mrs Whittaker's old medical records are delivered to the ward. Letters confirm that Professor Raymont, who had met Mrs Whittaker in clinic a few months earlier, considered her to have pseudo-seizures on a background of bipolar disorder. He had recommended recommencement of lithium which Mrs Whittaker had stopped taking some years prior. The letter mentions that Mrs Whitaker was seen with her husband, who is variously described as supportive, caring and attentive.

## What would you do?

Given this interesting presentation and emerging evidence of a psychiatric history, Dr Wallace elects to discharge Mrs Whittaker and asks the nursing staff to send her to the discharge lounge until her husband can come and collect her. Simultaneously he telephones the GP practice to see if there is any additional medical or social history of which he should be aware. The practice receptionist described the file as very thin and says that there does not appear to be anything out of the ordinary. The duty doctor is currently with a patient and cannot be disturbed.

Whilst Dr Wallace is on the telephone, his consultant comes to the ward. Mrs Whittaker approaches him in tears and states that she cannot go home. She is concerned that her husband will physically or sexually assault her, telling him that this has happened frequently of late, before lifting up her blouse to reveal multiple bruises over her flank.

---

*Avoiding Errors in Adult Medicine*, First Edition. Ian P. Reckless, D. John M. Reynolds, Sally Newman, Joseph E. Raine, Kate Williams and Jonathan Bonser.
© 2013 John Wiley & Sons, Ltd. Published 2013 by John Wiley & Sons, Ltd.

## What options are available to the consultant at this point?

### ⚖ Expert opinion

At this point, any doubts about the veracity of Mrs Whittaker's story should be put to one side. Sufficient concerns have been raised to warrant further action even if her account turns out to be fabricated. The presence of medically unexplained symptoms may be associated with abuse.

Dr Wallace and the rest of the team should focus upon the protection of Mrs Whittaker, pending further assessment. She should remain in hospital for the time being and it may be appropriate to move her so that her precise location cannot be determined by her husband.

The team's approach should have three elements: protection, information gathering and escalation of concerns to the appropriate professional or body.

In relation to protection, the team should contact the duty social worker and the Trust's lead for safeguarding adults in order to obtain further advice.

Information gathering will involve determining whether Mrs Whittaker, or indeed Mr Whittaker or anybody else living at the home address, is on the local authority's vulnerable adult register. A discussion with the relevant GP may also prove useful: is there a history of other episodes suggestive of abuse; does Mr Whittaker indeed have dementia and behavioural challenge; does Samantha live with her parents and how is their relationship?

Mrs Whittaker should be encouraged to see a social worker and if she does decide to leave before her full assessment, contact details for support should be provided to include specialized police teams and any local refuge for victims of domestic violence.

It should be noted that at this point in time, the confidentiality of the doctor–patient relationship can be set aside to a degree. The priority now is ensuring the protection and safety of all members of the family going forward.

### ⚖ Legal comment

Every NHS Trust has a vulnerable adult lead and a safeguarding policy for adults. It is also likely to be part of a local multi-agency agreed response network. A vulnerable adult is a person aged 18 years or over who is unable to take care of themselves or protect themselves from being exploited or harmed. This may be because they have a mental health problem, a disability, a sensory impairment, because they are old and frail or have some form of illness. Mrs Whittaker falls into the category of vulnerable adult.

If she has capacity then the safeguarding concern should be discussed with her. If she does not have capacity then there is a duty to act in her best interests in accordance with the local safeguarding protocol. If her daughter Samantha is still an inpatient, it would be acceptable, as part of the wider best interests information gathering, to ask for information about her parents' relationship and her mother's recent medical history.

Abuse is a violation of the individuals civil or human rights by another person or persons. It may consist of a single or repeated act. There may be an act of neglect or an omission to act, or it may occur when a vulnerable person is persuaded into a transaction to which he or she has not consented or cannot consent. Abuse ranges from treating someone with a lack of respect to causing actual physical harm. Abuse can be physical, sexual, psychological/emotional, financial or material and includes domestic abuse.

Physical abuse is physical harm caused deliberately by rough or thoughtless behaviour. Sexual abuse is making somebody do something of a sexual nature that they do not want to do or cannot consent to. Psychological or emotional abuse is behaviour that makes the individual feel anxious, intimidated or frightened, including verbal abuse, demeaning or threatening behaviour. Financial or material abuse is theft, fraud or exploitation putting pressure on an individual to use their money in a way that they do not want to or is not in their best interests.

Mrs Whittaker alleges that her husband spends the weekly household keeping as he wishes. If so, this may lead to her neglect, by failing to meet her physical care needs (for example withholding necessities such as adequate food and water, medicines and heating).

As the consultant is worried, he should document his concern and record any physical injury – in this case the severity of the bruising-in the healthcare records. If Mrs Whittaker has capacity he should discuss his concerns with her and seek her permission to take action. The consultant should make an adult protection referral to the local social services and if serious harm is suspected, he should also, report the matter to the police. Mrs Whitaker is making allegations of physical and sexual assault and, as the Consultant is aware that she has multiple bruises, this case does raise a suspicion of serious harm and so it should be referred to the police and social services.

There are local arrangements for adult safeguarding and a safeguarding adults board. There are likely to be county-wide codes of practice for the protection of vulnerable adults from abuse, exploitation and mistreatment. The safeguarding adults board is responsible for creating a framework within which all responsible agencies in the county work together to ensure a coherent policy for the protection of vulnerable adults at risk of abuse and a consistent and effective response to any circumstances giving ground for concern, formal complaints or expressions of anxiety.

It is likely that the local safeguarding adults board also have a policy statement on the criteria for the use of Independent Mental Capacity Advocates (IMCAs) who were introduced following the introduction of the Mental Capacity Act 2005.

### Patient confidentiality

There is a legal obligation on doctors to keep confidential what a patient tells them; but this obligation is not absolute. There are situations where the law obliges doctors to breach confidentiality and there are also situations where the law allows doctors to breach confidentiality. The General Medical Council provides professional guidance on this topic and although it does not have the force of law, it is taken seriously by the courts. There is no breach of confidentiality if a patient gives consent or cannot be identified. Sharing information about patients with other members of the Healthcare Team for the purpose of providing treatment is not generally viewed as a breach of confidentiality. There are a number of situations (for example, where the public health is at risk) when the law imposes a duty on doctors to disclose specific information to third parties. The GMC guidelines advise doctors who are asked to release information to weigh the possible harm both to the patient and to the overall trust between the doctor

and the patient against the benefits likely to arise from the release of information. For example, disclosure to an appropriate person in authority may be desirable for the prevention or detection of a serious crime. Serious crime in this context, is defined as a crime which will put someone at risk of death or a serious harm which would include abuse of a vulnerable adult.

### Discharge of patients who are clinically fit and refuse to be discharged

The legal duty on the hospital is to provide treatment to the patient until they are clinically fit for discharge from the acute hospital environment to a more appropriate setting; whether this be home with community support or to a nursing home or a care home. The grounds for Mrs Whittaker's refusal are that she is seeking to distance herself from domestic abuse. It is likely that if discharge is to a place of safety suitable for her current psychological/care needs whilst investigations are undertaken, then Mrs Whittaker will consent.

There is usually a Trust policy on discharge and transfer of care and a multi-agency cooperation agreement to provide either supported placements at home or suitable accommodation. When a patient who is clinically fit resists discharge, a meeting has to be convened to discuss the next steps. The measures available to the Trust are to charge the patient for the bed space and even (although rarely used) to obtain a possession order on the bed. Difficulties with patient discharge are usually the result of family disputes or lack of assistance from another public agency.

---

### ⚠️ Key learning points

**General points**

- Doctors must always be on their guard with respect to the possibility of abuse.
- The obligation placed upon doctors to maintain patient confidentiality is not absolute.

# Case 34 Funny turn

One morning, the medical registrar on-call is asked by the Emergency Department to see a 46-year-old motor sports journalist, Greg Dillon, after an episode of speech disturbance (expressive dysphasia) followed by a loss of consciousness. Mr Dillon's wife had given him jam and dextrose tablets although no blood sugar had been measured. It took over an hour for Mr Dillon's conscious level and speech to return to normal. He has now recovered completely but has a frontal headache.

Mr Dillon is a type 2 diabetic and takes once daily insulin and twice daily gliclazide. His blood pressure is well controlled, having been switched from a beta blocker to an ACE inhibitor two weeks prior because of erectile dysfunction. He smokes around ten cigars per week. He has been busy at work over the last few weeks in the run up to the British Grand Prix.

Examination is normal, as is a 12 lead ECG.

## What is your differential diagnosis?

Given the speech disturbance, the registrar takes the view that this episode was likely to have been a transient ischaemic attack and arranges appropriate investigations including a same day MRI with vascular imaging. She warns Mr Dillon that he is unlikely to be able to drive for a month following a TIA.

## What do you think of the diagnosis and the advice?

When the investigations have been completed, the AMU Consultant reviews Mr Dillon without the notes (the registrar is occupied with another patient). Mr Dillon explains that he still has a headache and the consultant, taking into account a normal MR examination, suggests the diagnosis of migraine. He discharges Mr Dillon with advice to watch his diet, alcohol intake and stress levels. He says that Mr Dillon can drive, as long as he feels well.

## Do you agree with the consultant?

Three days later, Mr Dillon is involved in a road traffic accident. It transpires that his blood glucose had fallen to 2.2 mmol whilst he was behind the wheel. Blood tests in the Emergency Department reveal acute renal failure (creatinine 300, baseline 90–105). Following a full recovery, Mr Dillon complains to the hospital arguing that a failure to reach the correct diagnosis had resulted in loss of his no claims motor insurance premium.

## Expert opinion

The differential diagnosis for transient neurological impairment is broad and includes cerebrovascular disease, epilepsy, migraine and hypoglycaemia. The latter should always be considered in a patient taking a sulphonylurea or insulin. Loss of consciousness is very rare indeed in transient ischaemic attack (TIA) and it should not form part of an initial differential diagnosis of loss of consciousness. Both migraine and hypoglycaemia can present with focal neurological symptoms and signs but migraine would also be an unlikely cause of loss of consciousness. Hypoglycaemia may resolve relatively slowly following an oral sugar load.

A normal MRI scan does not exclude a diagnosis of TIA: approximately 50% of scans will show some diffusion-weighted change whilst the remaining 50% will not. The diagnosis of TIA therefore remains clinical.

In this case, there was inadequate consideration of the range of diagnostic possibilities. This error was compounded by the consultant taking into account only two pieces of information (transient symptoms which had provoked a TIA protocol MRI and the emergence of a headache) to reach his diagnosis.

When advising patients about driving, the DVLA medical guidance should be followed to the letter. Where a range of diagnoses remain on the differential, the most restrictive guidance should be applied until the diagnosis can be made more firmly.

*Avoiding Errors in Adult Medicine*, First Edition. Ian P. Reckless, D. John M. Reynolds, Sally Newman, Joseph E. Raine, Kate Williams and Jonathan Bonser.
© 2013 John Wiley & Sons, Ltd. Published 2013 by John Wiley & Sons, Ltd.

## ⚠ Legal comment

This case highlights the importance of good communication between colleagues, especially when working in a area of high throughput such as acute medical admissions. It also raises important issues about recording advice given to patients (including in the discharge letter to the GP).

In this instance, whilst two incorrect diagnoses were entertained (TIA and migraine), the correct diagnosis (hypoglycaemia) was not considered. TIA is the only one of these three diagnoses which the DVLA says entails no driving for a period. A patient who takes medication such as insulin is not required by DVLA to stop driving after a single episode of hypoglycaemia, unless he loses consciousness (as happened in this case).

If liability to Mr Dillon were established, then he would be entitled to compensation for any personal injury sustained in the car accident as well as the direct financial losses resulting from the failure to make an earlier diagnosis. This would include a claim for loss of earning and other direct pecuniary losses. There may also be adverse reputational damage—given Mr Dillon's occupation—due to the loss of his no claims bonus.

## ⚠ Key learning points

### Specific to the case

- The differential diagnosis of transient neurological disturbance is broad and it may not be possible to make a diagnosis with confidence.
- When loss of consciousness has occurred, TIA is a very unlikely cause.
- MRI in the aftermath of TIA will be normal in approximately 50% of cases, with subtle abnormalities (diffusion restriction) in the remainder.

### General point

- Physicians should ensure that discussions are documented and where possible, there are supplementary pieces of evidence attesting to communication.

# PART 3

# Investigating and dealing with errors

## 1  Introduction

Part 1 of this book looked at how adverse incidents and errors occur. Part 2 examined detailed examples of errors. This third part looks at the mechanisms in place to pick up and then respond to errors. Those mechanisms are operated by the organization providing the healthcare (i.e. the hospital Trust), the wider NHS (NHSLA), the professional regulatory system (GMC), and by the legal systems beyond the NHS (the coroner, the civil or criminal courts).

A doctor who makes an error may find himself the subject of investigation and attention from each or any of these bodies. For example, the doctors in the vincristine case referred to in Part 1 will have no doubt faced internal hospital investigations with a view to disciplinary proceedings as well as external legal scrutiny.

There was a police investigation and it led to a criminal trial. The death of the patient was reported to the coroner and an Inquest was opened. The family of the patient will likely have sued the hospital for damages for civil negligence. The case will also certainly have come to the attention of the GMC.

Rightly or wrongly, criminal trial and referral to the GMC will have primarily focused on how those individual doctors were to blame for what happened, and only secondarily on the defects in the system which may have contributed to the outcome.

This section gives an account of the working of these processes. We also give some practical advice. However, a doctor facing an investigation of any significance will need considerable legal and moral support, as we explain below.

## 2  How hospitals try to prevent adverse errors and their recurrence

The following are the main mechanisms for picking up errors. They are themselves subject to continuous review and discussion.

### Guidelines and protocols

Guidelines are systematically developed statements to assist clinicians to make appropriate healthcare decisions. They should be statements of best

*Avoiding Errors in Adult Medicine*, First Edition. Ian P. Reckless, D. John M. Reynolds, Sally Newman, Joseph E. Raine, Kate Williams and Jonathan Bonser.
© 2013 John Wiley & Sons, Ltd. Published 2013 by John Wiley & Sons, Ltd.

practice based on a review of the current evidence. They should summarize the key information on a topic and should be reviewed at agreed intervals to ensure that they remain up to date and have taken into account new developments. Guidelines may be national (for example, those produced by the National Institute for Health and Care Excellence, NICE), or they may be issued by local organizations and tailored to suit local conditions, populations and facilities. They aim to reduce variation in practice. They serve as a useful source of reference although they do not necessarily need to be followed to the letter.

The term 'protocol' suggests a more rigid set of statements allowing little flexibility and minimal variation. A protocol sets a precise sequence of activities to be adhered to in the management of a specific condition. However, in practice, the terms 'guidelines' and 'protocols' are often used interchangeably.

Guidelines and protocols may need to be adjusted to meet individual circumstances. Clinical judgement should always be used. However, any reasons for deviating from a guideline or protocol should be documented and discussed with a senior doctor.

Guidelines and protocols can help reduce errors by minimizing the need to rely on memory. They can be particularly useful in stressful situations. Online versions avoid problems of paper copies being lost and are easier to update. They can be particularly helpful for trainees and for doctors facing an unusual situation. A review of an adverse incident can highlight the need to create a new guideline for a particular condition in order to reduce the likelihood of an error recurring.

## Clinical audit

Clinical audit is the process of comparing current practice with a defined standard of best practice (which may be based on local, national or international guidelines). The audit cycle involves collecting data, comparing it with the defined standard and then identifying gaps, deficiencies in practice or areas for improvement. Changes should then be implemented and the audit repeated. Clinical audit should be a continuous process to ensure that standards are monitored on an ongoing basis with the overall aim of enduring quality improvement.

All hospitals should have clinical audit programmes with systematic mechanisms for developing audit priorities, engaging stakeholders, communicating results and implementing changes. In many institutions, regular audit meetings provide a forum for some or all of these activities.

The role of audit is to promote best practice, but in so doing it may identify areas of error. It is a key component of clinical governance and hence is a tool for minimizing harm as well as maximizing quality.

## Global trigger tools

Global Trigger Tools are a recent development which aims to measure the rate of harm in healthcare by structured retrospective case note review. A number of tools have been developed for use in the UK.

A systematic review of case notes is performed using a standardized template, looking to identify key 'trigger' events which serve as clues that harm may have occurred. The notes are then further examined to see if these events did indeed result in harm. The aim is to identify priority areas for patient safety improvements. A number of sets of case notes should be reviewed at regular intervals, so allowing improvements to be tracked over time.

The process is based on the idea that traditional voluntary incident reporting does not reliably occur and is estimated to identify only 5-10% of harm events; whereas trigger tools detect harm rates in excess of 30%.

The emphasis is on exploring systems rather than individuals. It is not used to identify details of specific events – other tools may be needed for this. The data is intended to help minimize harm within an organization and not for comparisons between organizations.

## Incident reporting

All NHS Trusts have systems to identify and manage risk. Staff members have a duty to report not just errors but also untoward events. They should be familiar with the appropriate reporting procedures. An 'untoward event' is defined more widely than an error in the NHS. It is, 'any unintended or unexpected incident which could have or did lead to harm for one or more patients receiving NHS funded healthcare.'

It can be seen that the definition covers 'near misses' as well as incidents which actually caused harm. Hospital policies may give examples (or a 'trigger list') to help staff identify an 'untoward event'. For example, nonclinical incidents would include slips, trips and falls, violence and aggression. Clinical incidents would include medication errors, hospital acquired infections, delays in treatment, consent issues, and the unexpected death of a patient. It is estimated that 10% of NHS inpatients experience an adverse incident.

While there will be minor variations between different NHS Trusts on how these reports are managed, the normal process would include these steps:

1. The staff member should verbally report the incident to the supervisor/line manager/ward manager or hospital bleep holder on duty at the time of the incident.
2. The staff member should then complete the NHS Trust's Incident Report Form; this form may be either paper-based or electronic. Most Trusts request that this form be completed shortly after an incident has occurred. NHS Trusts are increasingly using online forms which in theory should make incident reporting quicker, easier and more accessible.

3. There will then be some form of internal management review by managers of the clinical service and the corporate risk team; this normally has to be completed within a defined timeframe and includes the collation of witness statements (see Part 3 Section 8: The role of the doctor, for guidance on witness statement writing).

4. The incident will then be graded and, depending on the classification, further investigation may take place. A Root Cause Analysis (RCA) may be undertaken using one of a number of standardized methodologies. Particularly serious incidents may be categorized as a Serious Incident Requiring Investigation (SIRI), previously referred to as 'Serious Unto-ward Incident (SUI)' and these incidents need to be reported formally and externally. When investigating an incident, the view of a clinician not directly involved in the care of the patient is often useful. In some cases an external review will need to be commissioned.

5. Once the appropriate level/type of investigation has taken place and the key and contributory factors have been identified an action plan will be agreed to ensure that appropriate preventative actions are put in place.

6. The staff involved in the incident will be given feedback once the investigation has been concluded.

7. The action plan will then be monitored by the hospital Trust until completed.

Summary information from incident reports is transferred electronically to the National Reporting and Learning System of the NHS Commissioning Board, so as to create a national database. This allows trends to become apparent which may not be obvious at local level.

Some incidents must also be reported to external bodies. The hospital Trust policy should specify these, but examples are:

1. Untimely, unexpected and suspicious unnatural deaths should be reported to the coroner and/or police.

2. 'Never Events' should be reported to the NHS Commissioning Board. A 'Never Event' is a serious, largely preventable patient safety incident which should not occur if appropriate preventative measures had been implemented. An example is wrong site surgery.

3. An incident that could impact on liability/indemnity cover arrangements should be reported to the NHS Litigation Authority.

4. Incidents that could involve the safeguarding of either adults or children should be reported to the local Safeguarding teams.

5. Any fatal injury to employees or other people in an accident connected with Trust business should be reported to the Health and Safety Executive.

A shortcoming of reporting systems is a perceived reluctance by staff to complete forms, partly because they are time consuming, and partly because of concerns that the reporter will be blamed for the incident or be seen to have blamed other people. It is thought that there is significant under-reporting of harmful events.

## Whistleblowing

As well as having a policy requiring staff to report untoward incidents, all NHS Trusts should have a whistleblowing policy, designed to protect an employee who wishes to raise any kind of concern about the operation of the Trust, including those relating to clinical matters. The policy will direct the employee to the appropriate manager to whom the concern should be expressed. The policy will require that manager to take the disclosure seriously and to investigate it as soon as possible. The policy will set timescales for responses and it will, if appropriate, feed into the incident investigation policy. The policy will make it clear that a whistleblower with a genuine concern will be protected from any kind of retribution or unfavourable treatment as a result of his disclosure, unless the whistleblower is found not to have acted in good faith, but to have raised a concern out of malice or when he knows the facts to be untrue.

Whistleblowing policies are based on the protection afforded by the Public Interest Disclosure Act 1998. The point of the Act (which should be reflected in any policy) is to encourage disclosures, so long as they are made to the appropriate person. A person who wants to blow the whistle in public (for example, by going to the media) may not be protected unless he has attempted to get his concern investigated internally, but has been ignored, or unless there is good reason to believe he would suffer if he raised it internally. Even then, it has to be an exceptionally serious matter for the protection of the Act to apply.

In January 2012 the GMC published new guidance for doctors about whistleblowing called "Raising and Acting on Concerns about Patient Safety" It is significant in that it places a positive professional duty on a doctor to raise concerns when he believes that patient safety is being compromised. In addition, it stipulates that a doctor must not enter into agreements with employers which restrict him from raising concerns about patient safety. A doctor who finds himself under pressure to sign such an agreement must point out his professional duty not to do so.

Advice about whistleblowing can be obtained from charities such as Public Concern at Work or from Trade Union representatives.

## Professional appraisal

All consultants and career grade doctors are required to undergo an annual appraisal. Trainees undergo similar assessments and appraisal through the Annual Review of Competency Progression (ARCP) process. The detail of appraisal should be private and confidential between the doctor and their trained appraiser. Appraisal is based on the GMC's 'Good Medical Practice' which describes the principles of good medical practice, and the standards of competence and conduct required of doctors in their professional work. The appraisal requires doctors to reflect upon their achievements and failings in the previous year and to consider what they would like to accomplish in the forthcoming year. As well as dealing with issues such as the doctor's clinical performance and effectiveness over the previous year, the appraisal should also deal with complaints (which should be reflected on and learnt from), disciplinary matters, probity, health, continuing medical education and audit. The appraisal landscape is currently in a state of flux on account of the introduction of the revalidation process (which will be underpinned by appraisal). This process is likely to result in appraisal that is more transparent, evidence rich and formalized. In most NHS organizations, the medical director has become the 'responsible officer', a lynchpin of the revalidation system.

Over recent years a new type of assessment called a 360 degree appraisal has also been performed in some hospitals alongside the standard appraisal. This appraisal involves anonymous feedback on a doctor's performance from 10–15 colleagues – doctors, nurses, administrative staff, managers and others. Anonymous feedback may also be obtained from patients using standardized forms. This type of appraisal is regarded by many consultants as being useful and complementary to the standard appraisal process. In time, it may become incorporated into the standard appraisal process.

## 3   The role of hospital staff

A significant part of hospital administration is involved with risk management and with the consequences of errors. The main roles/departments are as follows:

### Medical director

By law every NHS Trust has a medical director. This is a senior doctor who is responsible for the standard of medical care within the organization and for ensuring that relevant standards are met, for example: making sure patient confidentiality is protected and that medical equipment is checked and monitored.

The medical director is also responsible for doctors working for the Trust: for their work contracts, for supporting them in their continuing professional development, especially if they get into difficulties. The medical director is also likely to be appointed as the GMC's responsible officer for revalidation (see Part 3 Section 7: External investigation of errors and incidents—the GMC in future).

### Clinical director

The clinical director provides leadership within the department that he heads. In some organizations, the clinical director will also carry managerial and financial responsibilities whilst in others these reside with a general manager. The Clinical Director has a key role in investigating incidents and in ensuring that staffing, policies and practice are fit for purpose.

## Occupational health

The occupational health department aims to promote and maintain the highest degree of physical, mental and social well-being for all workers in the organization. The department leads on the prevention of work-related health problems; the protection of workers in their employment from risks; the placing and maintenance of the worker in an occupational environment adapted to his physiological and psychological capabilities; and, as summarized by WHO, 'the adaption of work to man and of each man to his job'. The occupational health doctor may have a role in investigating certain clinical errors where it is thought that they stem from a doctor's health problems.

## PALS

The Patient Advice and Liaison Service, known as PALS, has been introduced to ensure that the NHS listens to patients, their relatives, carers and friends, and answers their questions and resolves their concerns as quickly as possible.

In particular, PALS will:

- provide information about the NHS and help with any other health related enquiry;
- help resolve concerns or problems;
- provide information about the formal NHS complaints procedure and how to get independent help;
- improve the NHS by listening to patient concerns, suggestions and experiences and by ensuring that people who design and manage services are aware of the issues that have been raised;
- provide an early warning system for NHS Trusts and monitoring bodies by identifying problems or gaps in services and reporting them (NHS PALS website) http://www.pals.nhs.uk/

Whilst PALS has an independent air, staff members are typically employees of the NHS Trust.

## Legal services

Most Trusts will have a legal department to provide a comprehensive legal service to the Trust and its employees on any matter relating to hospital Trust business.

The main areas of responsibility are litigation (clinical and nonclinical), employment law, contract law, corporate law, procurement law and estates. The teams usually manage all cases referred to the coroner and also many issues where the court services or police are involved. In addition, a legal team is usually available during working hours to provide advice on any matter of a legal nature which relates to the hospital Trust's business. There will also be specific arrangements in place for obtaining urgent legal advice out of hours.

The most common day to day requests from doctors relate to consent and best interests, capacity (MCA 2005 and Deprivation of Liberty Safeguards), confidentiality (Data Protection Act 1998), providing information to third parties and the Freedom of Information Act 2000.

## Communications department

Communications departments are usually involved in raising the profile of Trusts, maintaining public and internal websites, writing staff newsletters and magazines, managing press enquiries, publicizing big events and major projects within the Trust and producing the annual report and other corporate documents. They will also be involved in managing any media interest after an adverse incident. Calls from local newspapers should be directed to them.

## Clinical governance

Clinical governance has been defined as 'a system through which NHS organizations are accountable for continuously improving the quality of their services and safeguarding high standards of care by creating an environment in which excellence in clinical care will flourish' (Scally and Donaldson, 1998, p. 61).

It is usually the clinical governance team in a hospital which ensures that all Executive Directors, commissioners and other appropriate authorities and stakeholders are informed of incidents. This may include the Care Quality Commission, Monitor (in the case of NHS Foundation Trusts), the Health and Safety Executive, the NHS Litigation Authority and the police.

## Risk management

Risk management departments have oversight of the whole spectrum of things that can go wrong. This includes slips, trips and falls involving staff, patients and the public, administrative errors that impact on patient care and clinical incidents that have a direct effect on the outcome of patient care.

## 4  The role of external agencies

There are a number of external agencies that play a role in the management of risk and incidents within NHS organizations. The National Patient Safety Agency was abolished in 2012 and its functions passed to other organizations as described below. The National Reporting and Learning System (NRLS) which collates information about clinical incidents from organizations across the NHS passed from the NPSA to the NHS Commissioning Board.

## NHS Litigation Authority (NHSLA)

The NHSLA plays two main roles in the management of risk in the NHS:

1. Clinical Negligence Scheme for Trusts (CNST), provides incentives to NHS Trusts to manage clinical risk actively through the development and implementation of appropriate policies, procedures and training. High performing NHS Trusts can receive a discount of up to 30% on their annual CNST premium (see Part 1, Section 1: Evidence from the NHSLA database).

2. National Clinical Assessment Service (NCAS), which supports the resolution of concerns about the performance of individual clinical practitioners to help ensure their practice is safe, comes under the auspices of the NHSLA from April 2013.


## National Clinical Assessment Service

NCAS was established in 2001. Its purpose is to advise healthcare organizations (both NHS and private) which have concerns about the practice of doctors, dentists or pharmacists for whom they are responsible. Its aim is to help those organizations look into questions about performance or conduct of a doctor quickly and fairly.

A person with authority at the organization (often, but not always the medical director) can telephone an NCAS adviser who will then talk through a case and advise on how to investigate further, whether to consider excluding a doctor and/or whether to implement disciplinary procedures. Advice given on the telephone will usually then be confirmed in writing. (Copies of correspondence will, in principle, be disclosable to the doctor under the Data Protection Act 1998.) As the case develops, the NCAS adviser will continue to advise as required by the organization. NCAS reported that over the first ten years of its existence, requests for help increased tenfold from about 100 in its first year, to more than 1000 in 2010.

In addition to advising, NCAS will, upon request, provide clinical assessment services. An assessment of a doctor's competence cannot be carried out without his agreement. (The idea will often be presented to him as the alternative to something that might be perceived as 'worse', e.g. disciplinary proceedings or a GMC referral.) An assessment might be directed towards clinical concerns, health concerns, 'communicative competence' and/or behaviour concerns. NCAS reports that about one referral in 20 will involve a full clinical assessment. Its published statistics show that general medical specialties account for 8% of referrals to NCAS and 7% of the full clinical assessments conducted. Older practitioners are more likely to be assessed than younger ones.

The clinical assessment process is wide-ranging and includes an occupational health assessment, a behavioural assessment, and a clinical assessment visit. There will be assessment workbook exercises and feedback from patients and peers.

The assessment will conclude with a report setting out the findings based on triangulated evidence (i.e. evidence from three different sources) and recommending the next step for both the doctor and the referrer. This will usually be a structured action plan, involving the monitoring of the doctor's performance with clear points identified at which the situation is to be reviewed.

In 2010/11, the assessment process ended with three out of every four practitioners assessed continuing to do clinical work, albeit nearly half of them with some kind of restriction on their practice.

In some cases of serious concern, there may be communication by NCAS and the referring Trust with the GMC. Advice may be given by NCAS on referring a case to the GMC.

From the doctor's point of view, the drawback to NCAS is that its advice is based only on what it is told by the referring organization. NCAS does not conduct its own investigation into matters save when a clinical assessment is requested. Furthermore, once its advice has been given, a Medical Director is highly likely to feel professionally obliged to follow it. Yet, because it is only advice, a doctor has no legal recourse against NCAS.

## The Healthcare Quality Improvement Partnership (HQIP)

The Healthcare Quality Improvement Partnership (HQIP) was established in April 2008 to promote quality in healthcare, and in particular to increase the impact that clinical audit has on healthcare quality in England and Wales. It is led by a consortium of the Academy of Medical Royal Colleges, the Royal College of Nursing and National Voices (formerly the Long-term Conditions Alliance).

## The Care Quality Commission

This body was established in 2009. Its purpose is to ensure that health and adult social care services are meeting the required standards. It does this through registration procedures and through inspections, which can be unannounced. It covers diverse services including hospitals, dentists, ambulances, care homes, family planning and slimming clinics. From 2012 its aegis has extended to primary medical services and it is planned that from 2013 GPs will also be required to register.

## Benchmarking

A number of organizations analyse routine data relating to health services in order to provide comparisons of the quality of care between different providers. These data are submitted by NHS Trusts through Hospital Episode Statistics (HES) to the Secondary Users Service (SUS). Data are anonymized at the patient level. The most prominent organization processing and presenting these data is Dr Foster Intelligence which produces the annual Hospital Standardised Mortality Rate (HSMR) and provides benchmarking information in relation to mortality, length of stay and readmission for a wide variety of conditions. CHKS is another major provider of risk adjusted outcome data. Such data frequently provoke an NHS Trust to examine a particular area of practice where that organization has been noted as a statistical outlier.

## 5   Hospital investigations

### Complaints management

A complaint is defined as 'an oral or written expression of dissatisfaction from an individual(s), which requires a response' (The Local Authorities Social Services and NHS Complaints (England) Regulations 2009).

Every NHS organization must have a formal written complaints procedure. The NHS Constitution sets out the various rights of the NHS patient. In particular all patients have the right to:
- have their complaint dealt with properly;
- know the outcome of any investigation into their complaint;
- local resolution by way of a patient meeting;
- take their complaint to the Parliamentary and Health Service Ombudsman if they are not satisfied with the way the NHS has dealt with it.

All NHS Trusts have, by virtue of the Health Act 2009, a duty to have regard to the NHS Constitution.

The overarching NHS Complaints Procedure requires:
1. all complaints to be registered and allocated a reference number; this will be done by the Complaints Department;
2. an acknowledgement to be sent within three working days;
3. all staff involved in the alleged incident to be asked to comment;
4. the Complaints Department to agree a response time with the complainant; this is usually a written response within 25 working days, or longer if agreed with the complainant;
5. in appropriate cases, a meeting is to be arranged with the complainant.

### Root cause analysis

This is the name given to a common sense method of investigation. Serious Incidents Requiring Investigation (SIRIs) should be examined through Root Cause Analysis. However the method can be used for investigating all incidents and complaints. A SIRI is defined as an incident that occurred in relation to NHS funded services and care resulting in one of the following:
- unexpected or avoidable death of one or more patients, staff, visitors or members of the public;

- serious harm to one or more patients, staff, visitors or members of the public; this includes cases where life-saving or major surgical/medical intervention is required, where the incident causes permanent harm, shortens life expectancy or results in prolonged pain or psychological harm;
- a scenario which prevents or threatens to prevent a hospital's ability to continue to deliver healthcare services; for example, actual or potential loss of personal/organizational information, damage to property, reputation or the environment, or information technology failure;
- allegations of abuse;
- adverse media coverage or public concern about the organization or the wider NHS;
- one of the core set of 'Never Events' as updated on an annual basis and currently including:
  - wrong site surgery
  - retained instrument post-operation
  - wrong route for administration of chemotherapy
  - misplaced naso-gastric or oro gastric tube, not detected prior to use
  - intravenous administration of wrongly selected concentrated potassium chloride

In practice, the definition of a SIRI may be applied flexibly and will be influenced by commissioners and other key stakeholders.

The purpose of RCA is to objectively determine the underlying and contributory causes of patient incidents, thereby enabling staff and management to learn from and avoid similar incidents in the future. Its essence is to go deeper than apparent causes of events, and in particular to look at the influence of external factors, including human factors.

The steps of a RCA investigation are as follows:

1. information collection;
2. information organization, including the production of a simple and tabular timeline;
3. information analysis, including identifying care and service delivery problems, contributory factors, failed and missing systems and the production of recommendations.

RCA investigations should ideally not be undertaken by a single investigator, but by a team. NHS Trusts should provide training to those who are expected to perform an investigatory role.

## Disciplinary procedures

A possible consequence of committing an error (or, more likely, a series of errors) is an investigation under the hospital's disciplinary procedure, and in particular under the procedure for dealing with issues of capability.

A doctor's contract of employment with his NHS Trust will incorporate that Trust's disciplinary procedure for medical staff. Since 2005 every NHS Trust in England has been required to model its disciplinary procedure for doctors on the framework published by the Department of Health in 2003 called 'Maintaining High Professional Standards in the Modern NHS' (known as 'MHPS'). This framework was intended to cure the defects of the previous slow and cumbersome process, which involved a legal chairman and the instruction of lawyers on both sides. In particular, the old system often led to prolonged suspensions of doctors ('gardening leave') for months, sometimes even years.

The new procedure requires the Trust to involve NCAS at an early stage. The intention is to reduce the need to use disciplinary procedures at all. However, in some circumstances, NCAS will advise a Trust that a case should be treated as a disciplinary matter.

MHPS divides all disciplinary matters into two groups, those involving issues of capability and those of misconduct. Capability issues arise, according to MHPS, when an employer considers that there has been a clear failure by an individual to deliver an adequate standard of care or standard of management, whether through lack of knowledge, ability or consistently poor performance. Underlying these problems there may be a lack of team working skills, out of date practice or just plain incompetence.

Misconduct, on the other hand, is a category that is concerned with inappropriate behaviour. Where the misconduct has nothing to do with the practice of medicine, the doctor will go through the same disciplinary procedure as any other employee of the Trust. If, however, the misconduct alleged is associated with the practice of medicine (for example, if it is said that he lied to cover up medical mistakes, he was unnecessarily rude to patients or colleagues, or he had an inappropriate relationship with a patient), then it is a question of professional misconduct, and the special procedures for medical staff laid down in MHPS apply.

MHPS goes on to say that any concerns about capability or conduct relating to a doctor in a recognized training grade should be considered initially as a training issue and dealt with via the educational supervisor and college or clinical tutor. A disciplinary hearing for a doctor in training is therefore comparatively rare, especially a hearing about his capability.

An outline of the disciplinary procedure now applicable in both capability and conduct matters is as follows:

1. A case manager is appointed at the Trust who must decide initially whether the case needs to be dealt with formally or informally. The case manager must have had no involvement in the issues under investigation. Often the clinical director takes this role.

2. If the case manager wants to look at the case informally, then with the assistance of NCAS, solutions involving training and support may be considered. These are often sufficient measures, particularly to deal with capability cases.

3. If the case is considered to require formal action, then the case manager should appoint a case investigator. The case investigator is likely to be another doctor at the Trust, probably from a different discipline. Again, he should have had no previous involvement in the issues in the case.

4. In the meantime, the case manager must also consider whether the duty to protect patients means that the doctor in question should be excluded from work or his clinical duties should be restricted during the investigation. The case manager may also consider whether a referral to the GMC is required, even at this early stage.

5. A further measure which can be considered in serious cases is the issue of an 'alert letter' warning other Trusts and private employers that the doctor is under investigation.

6. The case investigator then conducts an investigation, usually by interviewing relevant staff members and/or patients. Sometimes an expert report is commissioned.

7. The doctor should be informed of the investigation, and the specific allegations or concerns which are under consideration. He should be copied into all the paperwork and given an opportunity to put his point of view to the investigator.

8. The case investigator then writes a report to the case manager making recommendations for the future management of the case.

9. The case manager then decides whether or not to hold a formal disciplinary hearing.

10. If there is to be a disciplinary hearing, then whether the issues are ones of capability or professional misconduct or a mixture of the two, the disciplinary panel must consist of three people, one of whom must be a medically qualified person not employed by the Trust (but appointed by the Trust). (The other two members will be from within the Trust.)

Most NHS Trusts' disciplinary procedures provide that a doctor may be represented before a disciplinary panel by a colleague or friend, but not by a lawyer. However, in view of the very serious consequences to a doctor of a dismissal by his Trust (it can make it potentially difficult for him to practise his profession at all, since the NHS holds a near monopoly on the practice of medicine), it has been suggested in a judgment from the High Court that in certain serious cases, it may well be a breach of the doctor's human rights not to allow him legal representation. Increasingly, therefore, NHS Trusts do agree to legal representation in individual cases.

However, the argument was recently considered by the Court of Appeal and rejected. It was held that a doctor's "human right" to practise his profession was not engaged in local disciplinary proceedings, so that his rights are limited to a hearing which is conducted in accordance with MHPS (which does not provide for legal representation).

The outcome of a disciplinary hearing will be recorded in a letter to the doctor. The Panel must say which allegations have been found proven, and give a brief account of its reasons. It must then go on to consider what disciplinary sanction to apply in the light of its findings, namely whether the doctor should be dismissed from his post or given a warning (oral or written) or whether no action is necessary. In cases where the doctor is dismissed, the

Trust is highly likely to then refer the doctor to the GMC for an investigation into his fitness to practise.

The rights of the dismissed doctor are to appeal under the Trust's internal appeal procedure. He can also take his case to the Employment Tribunal if he considers the dismissal has been unfair, or the result of discrimination on the grounds of race, sex or age. Proceedings in the Employment Tribunal must be issued promptly (i.e. within three months) of the dismissal.

Sometimes a disciplinary procedure can be settled by way of a Compromise Agreement between the doctor as employee and the Trust as employer. Such an agreement may be a way for the doctor to resign and avoid the stigma of a dismissal, agree the terms of a reference and any financial package. For the Trust, it may be a way to resolve potentially messy and expensive litigation.

## 6 Legal advice – where to get it and who pays

If, despite a doctor's best intentions and endeavours, he finds himself on the wrong end of a complaint or an investigation, such as we have described in this section, he may find himself catapulted from the more or less comfortable and familiar environment of the hospital ward into an alien, possibly hostile world, very different from his usual work experience. This is a world governed by legal rules, deadlines and procedures. The doctor will need assistance to guide him through this unfamiliar territory. Colleagues may offer advice and for more minor complaints, this may be enough. But if the complaint is at all serious, then he will require access to legal advice. For a complaint could be the beginning of a process which will end with limits on the physician's ability to practise, the payment of damages (which could even run to millions of pounds), and a requirement to pay the legal costs incurred by the patient and his family. Then there are the legal costs incurred by the lawyers representing the individual doctor or the clinical team. The level of these costs will usually be based on the time spent on the case, but bills of tens of thousands of pounds would not be unusual for a case of moderate complexity.

Who pays these legal bills? The answer depends on a number of factors that include the nature of the initial complaint, how it develops and in what capacity the treatment of the patient was provided.

### (a) NHS treatment

#### i Negligence claims
All doctors employed in NHS hospitals are covered for claims against them through the NHS mutual indemnity scheme the Clinical Negligence Scheme for Trusts (CNST), managed by the NHS Litigation Authority (NHSLA) in England. This means that the payment of both damages and all bills for legal advice in respect of claims will be organized through the NHSLA in England, Welsh Health Legal Services in Wales, the Individual Health Boards and Trusts in Northern Ireland and the Central Legal Office in Scotland.

These bodies will organize legal representation and make decisions about the conduct of the case. The doctors involved in the treatment of the patient will be expected to cooperate with the lawyers appointed by these public health bodies to defend the interests of the hospital Trust.

### ii Inquests and fatal accident inquiries

The hospital Trust will organize the provision of legal advice for its clinicians and other staff at an inquest if required. However, if there are conflicts between clinicians concerning the nature of the treatment leading up to a patient's death, then a physician may prefer to have his own legal representation at an Inquest, so that his individual care can be defended in an appropriate fashion. He cannot usually expect his own legal costs to be paid by the hospital Trust in those circumstances.

### iii Criminal inquiries

Sometimes a hospital Trust may pay for some of the initial defence costs of a criminal investigation. But this will depend on the nature of the case. The Trust may, for example, fund defence costs where the criminal charges arise from an apparent system failure. But the Trust may well conclude that the allegations are personal to the treating physician and should be dealt with by him. In general, criminal investigations will be personal to the clinician.

### iv General Medical Council

Complaints to the GMC will be considered personal to the physician. Accordingly, legal bills and the provision of legal services will not be covered by a hospital Trust.

### v Medical Defence Organizations

It is clear that circumstances may arise in which a doctor needs his own legal advice. This is where the Medical Defence Organization (MDO) comes to the doctor's aid.

Until recently there were only three indemnity organizations offering legal assistance to doctors in the United Kingdom, namely the Medical Protection Society (MPS), the Medical Defence Union (MDU), and the Medical and Dental Defence Union of Scotland (MDDUS). Now there are a number of other options, but these three organizations still look after the interests of the vast majority of UK clinicians. The terms of their cover vary from a type of insurance to discretionary cover, or a mixture of the two. To establish which cover is most appropriate, we strongly recommend that doctors contact the MDOs to find out their terms and what they mean in theory and practice.

Whatever their differences, in essence, the MDOs offer members professional and legal advice. If a doctor is a member of one of these organizations, then, subject to the terms of his cover, he can call on that organization to come to his assistance in his time of need. All the MDOs offer telephone helplines, whereby a clinician can talk to a Medico-Legal Advisor on professional matters of concern, small or large.

So, although physicians are automatically covered against expenses arising out of negligence claims incurred in their NHS hospital work, they still need MDO cover for private work and for support in disciplinary proceedings and criminal investigations. The MDOs will also advise on whether there is a need for personal legal representation at an inquest and if so, they will often provide it. It is important for physicians to remember that although their interests will often be aligned with those of their employer, this may not always be the case. NHS Trusts will primarily seek to defend their own reputation and not necessarily that of the individual clinician. All doctors are strongly advised to maintain their own professional indemnity cover, over and above the protection afforded to them through NHS indemnity.

### vi Private work

If a physician undertakes private hospital work, then he will also need MDO cover against all types of claim or complaint arising from this work.

We have used the word 'need'. Is this overstating the case? There was talk in the Houses of Parliament a few years ago about whether clinicians should be legally required to have their own indemnity cover, but there was no formal debate and no legislation was drafted or passed. So it is not compulsory (although most private hospitals make it a condition of its contract with a doctor). But is it a risk worth taking? If a complaint or legal claim comes your way, then the costs and the damages could be crippling and the stress considerable. MDO membership provides support and a measure of peace of mind to the clinician who is subject to a complaint or claim.

## 7   External investigation of errors and incidents

### The Parliamentary and Health Service Ombudsman (PHSO)

A Complainant may not be satisfied with the outcome of a formal complaint made to an NHS organization. In that case the hospital Trust will tell him of his right to ask the Parliamentary and Health Service Ombudsman to investigate. This is the last port of call for a person with a formal complaint about NHS services.

A complainant can only approach the Ombudsman when the local complaints procedure has been concluded. The function of the Ombudsman is, upon request, and at his/her discretion to investigate an alleged injustice or hardship caused by a failure in administration or service in the NHS.

If the Ombudsman takes on the case after initial consideration and screening (and she does not have to do so) she has powers to call for relevant documents to be produced. Arrangements may be made for the main protagonists to be interviewed. The interviewees will be sent copies of their interview notes. The hospital will be sent a copy of the draft report, and given the opportunity to comment on it. In practice, the report will go through several drafts before it is concluded.

The report will comment on the standard of care and service found in the particular case. The Ombudsman cannot require any specific steps to be taken to remedy any hardship. She can only make recommendations. However those recommendations do have a strong moral force, particularly given the power to 'name and shame'. Generally, apologies or explanations to the complainant and/or an ex-gratia payment will be recommended. The Ombudsman may suggest ways to improve the service found to be at fault. The Ombudsman has recently published a high profile report called 'Care and Compassion' reciting her findings at a number of NHS institutions following complaints about poor care for the elderly. It can be seen that, as resources in the NHS become increasingly stretched, the Ombudsman could play an important role in setting and maintaining standards of provision.

When the role of Parliamentary and Health Service Ombudsman was first established, consideration of questions of clinical judgement by an individual doctor were specifically excluded from her remit. This has subsequently changed, and so the Ombudsman can and does now comment on the clinical judgements made by individual doctors, especially when an issue is whether those judgements have led to injustice and hardship. The Ombudsman will usually appoint Independent Assessors from the relevant medical speciality to advise on such questions. The conclusion on such questions will be based both on the facts and on the relevant professional standards (in the case of doctors, the *Bolam* test as described in Part 1, Section 2).

Once concluded, the Ombudsman's reports are put before Parliament. They are also available on the Internet and are very much in the public domain. A doctor who is exposed to the risk of criticism in this report may be well advised to ask his MDO for support in corresponding with the Ombudsman before it is published. Once published, his only recourse is by way of Judicial Review in the High Court, which may possibly provide a remedy if the Ombudsman's reasoning is significantly flawed or she has exceeded her remit.

## Negligence claims and the litigation process

If a patient or a patient's family issues a claim against an NHS hospital about a doctor's care and clinical management then the NHSLA will instruct one of its panel solicitors to investigate the claim and to defend it, if that is appropriate. The NHSLA's panel solicitors in liaison with the Trust's Legal Department will deal with the day-to-day management of the case, responding to correspondence from the patient's legal team and attending procedural hearings at court. They will keep the Trust and, through the Trust's Legal Department, the doctor himself abreast of developments. One of the roles of the solicitor and of the Trust's Legal Department acting on behalf of a clinician is to support him and to minimize the worry for him.

In practical terms, a doctor's initial involvement will be to comment on the Letter of Claim and the Trust's draft Letter of Response. There may also be a meeting with the Trust's Legal Department or NHSLA panel solicitor to discuss his treatment of the patient. The Legal Department and/or the NHSLA panel solicitor will normally draft a statement summarizing that treatment and will ask the doctor to approve its contents. This will be used to obtain expert opinion on the case. The doctor will be sent the appropriate documents, such as the medical records, the family's statements, the reports of the experts for the Trust and those for the family. He will also be asked for comments on these documents.

If the case appears defensible, then the NHSLA will wish to test the evidence and will arrange a conference with Counsel, i.e. a meeting with a barrister either in person or by video-link. The doctor will normally be required to attend such a meeting. The barrister will question him closely on his treatment of the patient and ask the experts to comment on that treatment. It may be that the NHS legal team will need two or three conferences before a final decision is made to defend the case in court or to reach a settlement with the patient. In rough terms, it will probably take three years from the first notification of the claim until a case comes to trial. However, the vast majority of claims are settled before trial, in some cases because the Claimant withdraws or in others because the NHSLA makes an offer to settle.

Negligence claims make only a relatively small call on a doctor's time. The damages and costs payable to the patient come out of government funds, or from the coffers of an MDO if the patient was treated privately. Such claims do not attract any sanction in themselves to affect a doctor's ability to work as a doctor.

The NHSLA now requires annual risk management reports on clinical negligence claims from its panel solicitors and an annual assurance return from NHS Trusts that action plans are in place for organizational learning from claims where clinical risks have been identified. This could include the requirement for training or supervision of a doctor's practice.

## Coroner's Court

In England, Wales and Northern Ireland where there is a sudden death of which the cause is unknown, where there has been a violent or unnatural death, or where there has been a death in custody, the case has to be referred to the coroner for an inquest, or inquiry. (In Scotland, there is a different procedure, which we describe below).

The coroner's role is to answer four simple factual questions:-
1. Who died?
2. When did he or she die?
3. Where did he or she die?
4. How did he or she die?

In practice, it is the latter question that tends to occupy the coroner's time. When he explores this question, it is important to understand that, in principle, he is not allowed to ask questions which ascribe blame or responsibility. He should restrict himself to the bare facts. In practice, however, establishing how someone died often tends to raise just such questions.

The coroner will gather evidence from the key individuals involved. His enquiries will be assisted by the expert opinion of the pathologist who carries out the post-mortem examination. He may also seek other expert opinion, medical or nonmedical, to help him reach a conclusion.

If you are asked to assist a coroner's enquiry, you will be asked to provide a statement outlining your involvement. As this will be read not only by the coroner, but also possibly by the other witnesses, it may be important to seek advice about it. Your employing Trust's legal department and/or lawyers will usually be able to assist and advise you. Failing that, you should seek advice from your MDO.

Unless the coroner decides, having looked at the papers, that the death was, after all, a natural one which he has no duty to investigate, he will hold a public hearing by way of investigation (or inquest). Witnesses, including the doctors involved, may be called to give evidence.

The coroner's court is not like other courts. In theory, it is not an adversarial procedure, no one is on trial, there are no sides or parties, and no prosecution or defence. Instead, there are just persons with an interest in the proceedings. These characteristics are unique in the English legal system and of ancient origin. In practice, NHS Trusts and families may well be represented by lawyers, especially when a negligence claim or adverse publicity may follow.

The coroner runs the court. Thus all witnesses are called by the coroner and he asks them most of the questions. The coroner directs the case, which is driven by his opinion. In certain limited circumstances, such as a death in custody, a jury is required to hear the evidence and reach a verdict.

Others with an interest in the proceedings, such as the family or the hospital Trust, also get an opportunity to ask questions of witnesses. The coroner must ensure that only questions which are relevant to the Inquest are put to the witnesses, that is to say, relevant to the four factual matters he is required to investigate.

It is, however, sometimes the case that the family of the deceased feels someone or some organization (such as a hospital) is to blame for the death. They see the Inquest as an opportunity to explore and expose that fault. While, in principle, the coroner is not allowed to make findings of fault, the question 'how' someone died often does beg the question of fault. For example, if someone dies unexpectedly, the investigation may focus on how a delay in treatment contributed to the death. In addition, the coroner has the power to make a finding of 'neglect' in certain extreme cases of a total failure to provide basic care and attention when it was obviously required. The family may ask the coroner to make such a finding, for example, in a case where the patient was left waiting on a trolley for treatment for an unacceptably long time.

For a doctor, it is an obvious occupational hazard that a patient might die unexpectedly. If a doctor is only asked to attend an Inquest once or twice in his career, he will have been fortunate. He is likely to feel uncomfortable anyway, but especially if he knows the case is a contentious one. Normally, the doctor's employing hospital Trust would provide any legal representation considered necessary for all staff members who are giving evidence. But there may be circumstances when the Trust feels unable to provide representation for a particular doctor. Equally, a doctor may feel he cannot be confident his Trust will provide him with adequate legal support or he may feel he needs very particular support. In those cases, it may be appropriate for an individual doctor to have his own lawyer at the Inquest to look after his interests. The MDO will give advice on this situation, and if appropriate, will instruct a lawyer.

Having heard the evidence, the coroner (or perhaps the jury) will deliver his 'verdict'. Traditionally, this was limited to a short form verdict including death by natural causes, or accident or misadventure (which means an unintended consequence of an intentional act – an example would be a surgical mishap), suicide, unlawful killing or an open verdict (to name the most common). As already mentioned, the coroner might add a rider of 'neglect' to some verdicts. This is a finding a hospital will be at pains to avoid.

The coroner is also permitted, under Rule 43 of the Coroner's Rules as amended, to serve a 'Rule 43 Letter' on an NHS organization (or another party) with the aim of reducing the risk of future deaths and requiring the relevant authority to take action to prevent the reoccurrence of a similar fatality. When served with a Rule 43 Letter, the recipient Chief Executive of the NHS Trust has 56 days to make a response with evidence of organizational investigation, learning and action plan. Both the letter and the response are lodged with the Lord Chancellor and copied to the Ministry of Justice which publishes an annual report of all Rule 43 letters issued by coroners. The issue of a letter under Rule 43 will be noted by commissioners and healthcare regulators and may provoke further interest or action on their part.

Instead of the traditional brief verdict, there is now a trend for coroners to return a 'narrative verdict'. This is a short factual summary, usually only four or five lines long. It is meant to give a more satisfactory outcome to the hearing, which may have been an emotional trauma for the family, than the standard short form verdicts.

Inquests are held in public, and there are often reports of them in the local or even national press.

## Fatal accident inquiries

In Scotland, there is a different procedure for investigating the circumstances of a death. Under the Fatal Accident and Sudden Death Inquiry

(Scotland) Act 1976, the Procurator Fiscal has discretion to investigate any death which is sudden, suspicious, unexplained or which occurred in circumstances that give rise to serious public concern. Some investigations are mandatory, namely cases of death in custody or as a result of an accident at work. In a minority of these investigations, the Procurator Fiscal will call for a hearing, known as a Fatal Accident Inquiry. That hearing takes place before a Sheriff in the Sheriff's Court. Acting in the public interest, the Procurator Fiscal will present the evidence. Other interested parties may be represented by lawyers (and often are). The Sheriff must produce a determination establishing:

1. where and when the death took place;
2. the cause of death;
3. any reasonable precautions whereby the death might have been avoided;
4. any defects in the system of working which contributed to the death;
5. any other relevant circumstances.

Unlike the coroner's proceedings, questions of fault are very much at issue in these proceedings, which are often quite high profile.

## Criminal matters

Sometimes things can go very badly wrong. A patient or an NHS organization may make an allegation against a doctor of a crime, such as crimes of fraud, indecency or assault. A patient may die unexpectedly shortly after receiving treatment. In these cases, the matter is passed to the police to investigate.

Initially the police will take an overview. They will have to obtain evidence to support the allegation. This might be a post-mortem report, or if it is an allegation from a patient, then a statement from the patient concerned.

Then the police will want to speak to the doctor.

It cannot be stressed enough how important it is for the doctor to seek advice and assistance if he knows or suspects that there is or may be a police investigation.

The police do not have 'chats', even though that is what they might call it when they contact the doctor. In fact the doctor will be interviewed under caution and that discussion will be recorded.

Proper preparation for any interview with the police is vital. It is often said that cases are not won at the police station stage, but they can certainly be lost if the foundation of the doctor's case is insufficiently robust.

Preparation may include a second post-mortem. It will certainly include lengthy meetings between the doctor and his legal and medical defence team, to analyse in depth the doctor's recollection of events. In most cases, a statement will be prepared to help the doctor and act as an aide memoire in the interview. In many cases, the doctor will be advised to simply read the statement and answer no further questions.

The police station interview will, by the very nature of it, be an alien, unfamiliar and intimidating experience. It is not at all like it seems in television dramas. The police now have the power to arrest whenever they feel it is necessary. The doctor's definition of 'necessary' is likely to be different from theirs. In short, if a doctor is to be interviewed, he should anticipate that he may well be arrested just before hand.

At the start of the interview, the doctor will be 'cautioned'. This is the form of words used to ensure the police can record anything he says in answer to their questions. The words of the caution are, 'You do not have to say anything, but it may harm your defence if you do not mention when questioned something which you later rely on in court. Anything you do say may be given in evidence.' The effect of this is that the doctor's initial account must be as comprehensive as possible. The court could make adverse inferences about any future additions to his account, for example when he gives evidence at trial.

Thankfully, most police officers realize that doctors are busy professionals. They will try to arrange a mutually convenient time for him to attend the police station. However some officers are still fond of the 'dawn raid'. Even if this happens, the doctor is entitled to representation. He should try to contact his MDO, but if that fails there is always a duty solicitor available to assist in the first instance.

Following the interview, there will be a period of waiting. The police will have other enquiries and when they are complete they will have to seek advice from lawyers at the Crown Prosecution Service (CPS). The more complex the case, the more protracted the waiting. In the more complex manslaughter cases the waiting can even run to a couple of years.

The prosecution has to provide, so that the jury is sure of guilt, evidence both that the act happened and the mental element of the offence. The mental element is usually (but not always) that you intended to do what is alleged. However, the charge of Gross Negligence Manslaughter is slightly different. For this charge, the jury has four questions to decide

1. Was there a duty of care?
2. Was that duty breached?
3. Did the breach cause the death?
4. Was the negligence so 'gross' that it was criminal?

If everything goes well, the doctor will in due course be told that there is no further action. That is the end of the police investigation. However, the Trust could still investigate and that the police are very likely to pass their file to the GMC which will conduct its own investigation.

If it does not go well, the doctor will be charged. Whilst all criminal cases start in the Magistrates Court, those involving doctors are often more serious and so will be transferred to the Crown Court for trial. Any trial could be many months in the future. In the meantime, the employing trust and the GMC may each take action in the interim to restrict or suspend the doctor's licence to practise.

In any dealings with the police or courts, remember paragraph 58 of Good Medical Practice (GMP). This states:

> you must inform the GMC *without delay* [emphasis added] if, anywhere in the world you have accepted a caution, *been charged with* [emphasis added] or found guilty of a criminal offence . . .

However, and somewhat confusingly, the caution given at the beginning of an interview is different from the 'caution' one might receive from a minor offence. The GMC means the latter caution at paragraph 58 of GMP, not the caution given during the police interview.

If convicted of the offences of fraud, sexual assault or manslaughter, the risk of a prison sentence is high. However each case is dealt with on its own merits and thus imprisonment is not inevitable.

Thankfully, prosecutions are very rare and when they do occur, acquittal rates are high.

## Public inquiry

Public inquiries might take place where:
- there has been a widespread loss of life;
- there are threats to public health or safety;
- there is a failure of duty by a statutory body to protect individuals.

However, there is no definitive list of events that will trigger the need for a public inquiry. A single death can lead to an inquiry, such as was the case in respect of the death of Victoria Climbie. More commonly, an inquiry will be held in response to numerous deaths as was the case with the Bristol Royal Infirmary Inquiry and the Francis Inquiry into the Mid-Staffordshire NHS Foundation Trust.

The Chairman of a public inquiry has the power to require witnesses to give evidence upon oath and to provide documents. Anyone refusing to comply could be charged with a criminal offence. However, the Chairman has a duty to act fairly to witnesses. Accordingly, any witness who is at risk of being criticized in the report of the Inquiry should be warned of that possibility, ideally before he gives evidence. The Chairman should send that person a letter, setting out the potential criticism and the evidence which supports it. That person should be given an opportunity to respond to the criticism. A doctor who receives such a letter should certainly contact his MDO for assistance.

## General Medical Council in practice

There are now approximately 231 000 doctors registered with the GMC and subject to its regulations. The statutory purpose of the GMC set out in the current Medical Act of 1983 is to 'protect, promote and maintain the health and safety of the public by ensuring proper standards in the practice of medicine'.

Over recent years GMC Fitness to Practise Procedures have been substantially reformed. Figure 3.1 outlines GMC processes. These reforms were designed to reassure the public in the wake of some well publicized scandals that concerns about substandard doctors are being dealt with efficiently and promptly. The most recent reform, introduced in June 2012, is the creation of the Medical Practitioners' Tribunal Service. This body is part of the GMC, but is described as operationally separate from it. Its function is to run the various Panel hearings, so that the adjudication of cases is demonstrably separate from the investigation and prosecution of cases by the GMC.

Most complaints to the GMC are from members of the public, but a substantial minority come from a public health body or from the Police. In the case of a referral by the Police or the doctor's employing hospital Trust, it is likely to be the result of an investigation or criminal procedures, and the doctor will probably have been told of the referral. In the case of a patient complaint, though, the doctor might well be taken by surprise when he receives a letter from the GMC.

We will now explain what that letter from the GMC may contain, its potential consequences and what the doctor needs to do to protect himself.

## Nature of the letter and the complaint

A doctor will find enclosed with the letter from the GMC a copy of the initial complaint. The letter itself will inform a doctor that the GMC are starting to investigate the complaint.

The variety of circumstances that might lead to a GMC referral are, of course, infinite and can touch on any aspect of practice, not just clinical judgement. Often the complaint will refer to a poorly conducted medical investigation and to a bad outcome from treatment. But other common complaints relate to a doctor's health, i.e. that poor mental or physical health is impairing his ability to practise effectively, to dishonesty (such as false claims on a CV, failure to disclose a conviction, altering medical records), to affairs with patients or to criminal investigations (fraud, sexual assault, drink driving).

The letter will also invite the doctor to comment on what the complainant has to say. He should get advice from his MDO on whether to send a response. He may be anxious to put his side of the story as soon as possible, but it is not always wise to do so at this early stage.

## Case investigation

The GMC has a service target of six months for concluding its investigations. So, after the initial letter, it could be some time before the doctor hears again. If on completing their investigations, the case managers decide to proceed with the case, then the results of the investigation will be presented to the doctor in a further letter, accompanied by a bundle of documents. This is known as a 'Rule 7 letter'. It sets out a series of allegations and the doctor will be asked to comment in writing before the Case Examiners decide what course of action to take. The doctor's reply to the Rule 7 letter is his major opportunity to persuade the GMC's Case Examiners that the allegations are unwarranted and that the case should be dropped at this preliminary stage.

The doctor is likely to feel very strongly about the allegations and the temptation is to express himself in emotional language. But this would be a mistake. Florid language may be taken by the GMC as evidence that he lacks insight. This is the cardinal sin. His response should be dispassionate and reasoned. He is therefore, strongly recommended not to write this letter himself, but to take advice from his MDO on what his strong or weak points are and on how to phrase his response.

## Interim orders

In a significant minority of cases, the doctor will be informed in the initial complaint letter that the GMC's Case Examiners have decided to refer the matter to the Interim Orders Panel (IOP) and that there will be a hearing in a few days to decide whether interim restrictions (such as suspension) should be imposed on the doctor's registration, while the case is being investigated. The doctor will be invited to attend that hearing, which will be held in Manchester, to present his arguments as to why no order should be made.

A doctor who receives such a letter should contact his MDO without delay and arrange to see an advisor. He will also need time off work to attend the hearing itself.

The Interim Orders Panel has the power to restrict a doctor's ability to work when it thinks, on the basis of the complaint made, that his fitness to practise *may* be so badly impaired that he poses a risk to the public. In general, the kinds of cases referred to IOP are those where there are significant performance concerns, or where the doctor is accused of misconduct involving impropriety or a lack of probity, for example, altering medical records or presenting a false CV. Generally, the IOP will be slow to suspend a doctor when the allegations have not been tested and are unproven. They will prefer to impose conditions allowing him to continue to practise. Interim conditions will usually involve safeguards such as supervision, mentoring or restrictions on the kind of work he can do. Allegations of lack of probity are more likely to meet with an interim suspension, since no conditions are considered adequate to protect the public from a deceitful doctor.

In principle, an interim order will last for 18 months (with reviews every six months), which is the time considered sufficient for the GMC to investigate the case and, if necessary, hold a Fitness to Practise hearing.

Given the potentially serious consequences of a suspension or of conditions being imposed, it is clearly in the doctor's interests to have a good legal team representing his interests at the initial hearing. This should be organized by the medico-legal advisor at his MDO.

## The Case Examiners

The doctor's Rule 7 response, along with the GMC's bundle of papers is then put before two Case Examiners (one medical and one lay). Their task is to consider whether on the available evidence there is a realistic prospect of establishing that his fitness to practise is impaired. If not, a number of options are available. They can close the case, issue a letter of advice, or invite the doctor to accept a warning on his registration. In cases covering health or poor performance, they can invite the doctor to accept certain undertakings. If however they think there is a realistic prospect of proving impaired fitness to practise, then they must refer the case to a Fitness to Practise Panel for a hearing.

## Performance assessments

Complaints suggesting a pattern of poor performance may lead to a direction that the doctor's performance be assessed by a specially appointed team. He will have his knowledge and competence tested objectively in various tests (knowledge tests and OSCE), and also subjectively in interviews with him and with his colleagues. A detailed report will then describe what areas of his practice are found to be acceptable, cause for concern or unacceptable. The assessors will conclude with an overall finding on whether his performance is deficient, and if so the steps they recommend to remedy those deficiencies. This report will form part of the Case Examiners' investigations and may then be the basis for either agreeing undertakings or making a referral to a Fitness to Practise Panel.

## The decisions of the Case Examiners

In the majority of the cases that come before them, the Case Examiners decide not to take any further action or to simply send a letter of advice to the doctor. But they can also issue warnings or invite undertakings. The most serious cases will, however, proceed to a hearing before a Fitness to Practise Panel. In 2010, the Case Examiners' decisions were as shown in Table 3.1.

## Warnings

A warning may be considered appropriate if the Case Examiners think the doctor's behaviour or performance has fallen significantly below the expected

**Table 3.1** Case Examiner decisions.

| | |
|---|---|
| Refer to Panel | 314 |
| Undertakings | 102 |
| Warning | 183 |
| Advice | 458 |
| Concluded (i.e. no further action) | 497 |
| **TOTAL** | 1554 |

standard, but not to such a degree as to indicate impaired fitness to practise. A common example would be drink driving. A warning will remain on the doctor's registration for five years but subsequently will still remain in the public domain, albeit marked 'expired'.

In practice, the doctor might have some limited opportunity to negotiate the wording of the proposed warning. However, if this outcome is unacceptable to him there is a right in some circumstances to challenge it before an Investigation Committee. In a significant number of cases, the Investigation Committee decides not to issue a warning after all.

## Undertakings

Undertakings are a set of written agreements restricting the doctor's practice. They are likely to comprise supervision arrangements and are usually appropriate in cases concerning a doctor's health or performance. They last indefinitely, until the Case Examiners in their discretion decide that they are no longer necessary.

If undertakings are accepted then, provided that they are not confidential, they are published on the doctor's registration for as long as they are current. Even when no longer current, the inquirer will still be able to find out about them, as part of a doctor's registration history.

If the doctor does not accept the undertakings, his case will be referred to the Fitness to Practise Panel with the threat of more severe sanctions including the ultimate penalty – erasure of his name from the register of practitioners.

## Referral to a Fitness to Practise Panel and erasure

The most common kinds of case referred to the Fitness to Practise Panel concern substandard treatment. In theory, a single clinical mishap should not be sufficient to establish impaired fitness to practise. What primarily concerns the GMC is a pattern of poor performance. But it does sometimes happen that a doctor with an otherwise excellent clinical reputation can find himself before a Panel because of one serious adverse case.

A Fitness to Practise Hearing is conducted in the manner of a criminal trial. At the start of the hearing, for example, the doctor is required to stand while the charges against him are read out by the Panel Secretary. Unless the hearing concerns confidential matters, such as those relating to the doctor's health, it will normally be in public. On the other hand, since 2008 the doctor no longer has the relative protection of the criminal standard of proof, 'beyond reasonable doubt'. Now the GMC prosecutors only have to prove the case on the lesser standard of 'on the balance of probabilities' (in other words, that the allegations are more likely to be true than not).

The hearing itself will usually take place in Manchester and will be before a Panel of at least three people (in longer cases, it should be five). Doctors in

**Table 3.2** FTP panel outcomes.

| | |
|---|---|
| Erasure | 73 |
| Suspension | 106 |
| Conditions | 37 |
| Undertakings | 5 |
| Warning | 29 |
| Reprimand | 0 |
| Impairment – no further action | 4 |
| No impairment | 65 |
| Voluntary erasure | 7 |
| **TOTAL** | 326 |

this situation are often surprised that only one member of the Panel must be a doctor, and even then, not necessarily from the same speciality.

At the end of the hearing, the Panel will decide:

1. whether (unless they are already admitted) the charges against the doctor are proven;
2. whether the charges which are admitted or found proven are sufficient to establish that his Fitness to Practise is impaired (whether by reason of misconduct, deficient performance or ill health); and
3. if so, what sanction is appropriate for the protection of the public. The sanction can range from a reprimand to conditions or suspension or the ultimate sanction of erasure from the register. Once erased, a doctor cannot apply to be restored to the medical register for at least five years.

Even in cases where Fitness to Practise is found not to be impaired, the Panel can be asked to consider whether to impose a warning on the doctor's registration, as an indication of its disapproval of his conduct.

It is important to appreciate that when considering whether a doctor's fitness to practise is impaired, the Panel must look not just at past failings but also at the doctor's present and future fitness to practise. A doctor who can demonstrate he understands his past failings (i.e. he has insight) and has taken action to improve his performance (i.e. remediation) may well not be impaired after all. Table 3.2 shows the outcomes of Fitness to Practise Panels in 2010.

## A trainee physician under the spotlight at the GMC (based on a real case)

Dr A was working as an FY2 doctor on a night shift on the Acute Medical Unit, under the supervision of a Registrar. He took a call in the early hours from a doctor in the Emergency Department, requesting the admission to AMU of a patient with a differential diagnosis of PE, viral infection or anxiety. On the instructions of his Registrar, Dr A requested that a D-Dimer test be taken before transfer.

Dr A and his supervising Registrar later went to see the patient in the ED where Dr A clerked him and recorded his history and presenting condition in the notes. The patient's history was of a cough for four weeks. He had returned from Australia a week previously and now had shortness of breath and a tight chest. He was admitted to the AMU on the basis of Dr A's working diagnosis of hypotension, chest infection and acute renal failure.

Later that morning, Dr A assisted the consultant on a post take ward round. It was alleged that when asked for the result of the D-Dimer test, Dr A replied that it was 0.1 (a negative result). The consultant and Dr A then went to see the patient who was sitting up in bed, fully conscious with no shortness of breath. Clinical examination found the patient's lungs were clear, and there were no clinical signs of DVT. Arterial blood gases were normal. The consultant did not advise anti-coagulant medication because, provided with a D Dimer test result of 0.1, he discounted a possible diagnosis of pulmonary embolism.

However, later that day the patient had a cardiac arrest due to a pulmonary embolism, and subsequent died despite treatment in ITU. It became clear that in fact the result of the D-Dimer test was 2.77, consistent with the possible presence of a blood clot.

An inquest was held and Dr A provided a written statement to the coroner and gave oral evidence on oath.

In due course there was a hearing before the GMC's Fitness to Practise Panel, where Dr A admitted an allegation that he failed to follow up the D-Dimer test result at a time when it was his responsibility to do so.

It was also alleged that Dr A had provided inaccurate information to the consultant on the post take ward round about the D-Dimer test result. Dr A denied this. After considering his evidence and that of the Consultant, the Panel decided it preferred Dr A's evidence. The reason was that, looking at the various statements made by the Consultant (to the Trust, to the coroner and to the GMC), the Panel found that they varied and contradicted each other, despite being prefaced by comments such as, 'I vividly recall' and 'I clearly remember this conversation even now.'

It was also alleged against Dr A that when he saw the patient in the ED, he failed to adequately assess his condition. Dr A denied this and so the Panel compared the notes he had made with those already made by the ED doctor. The Panel found the similarities of phrasing and sequence were such that Dr A must have simply copied them without conducting his own examination. Furthermore, in copying them, he omitted any reference to the ED doctor's differential diagnosis of pulmonary embolism, even though he should have known it was a possibility. Accordingly the Panel found this allegation proved.

It was further alleged that when he provided a written statement to the coroner, Dr A failed to give a full account of his involvement in events and he had therefore been dishonest and/or misleading.

The Panel heard evidence that before writing his statement, Dr A had been provided with the hospital's 'Guidance on Writing a Statement'. This stated there was a requirement he covered 'all essential points'. The Panel found that, despite this, Dr A's statement omitted to mention that he knew a D-Dimer test had been requested, and omitted to say he had discussions with other doctors about a possible diagnosis of pulmonary embolism.

It particularly noted that Dr A's statement to the coroner used the expression 'On examination, I found the patient to be . . . '. Having already found that Dr A had simply copied the results of the previous examination in the ED, the Panel found this statement was dishonest.

In conclusion, in relation to the clinical issues, the Panel found that Dr A's failure to follow up the D-Dimer test result, his failure to adequately assess the patient and his failure to take into account the differential diagnosis of pulmonary embolus were each serious failings individually and even more serious when taken as a whole.

When considering his evidence to the coroner, the Panel found that Dr A had acted dishonestly which is, of course, a serious departure from the standards to be expected of a registered medical practitioner.

The Panel therefore concluded that Dr A's Fitness to Practise was impaired by reason of his misconduct.

The GMC's barrister then argued that the serious nature of the findings meant that Dr A should be erased from the medical register. Dr A's barrister argued that, as Dr A was a junior doctor at the time of the events, he was inexperienced in writing statements. In addition he had been under pressure from the Trust. His current employers had written letters reporting that Dr A was hard working, clinically sound and there were no issues with his integrity.

Weighing all these matters up, the Panel decided that the proportionate sanction was a 12 month suspension. They said they would hold a hearing to review his case towards the end of the period of suspension when they would expect to receive evidence from Dr A of how he had developed insight into the failings which had bought him to the attention of the GMC, of how he had kept his medical skills and knowledge up to date and evidence of his good conduct during the period of suspension.

## The GMC in future

Two significant developments in the GMC's procedures are ongoing.

### (a) Revalidation

This concept has been much discussed since the Shipman Inquiry highlighted what has been termed 'a regulatory gap' between a doctor's employer and the GMC.

> Some doctors [are] judged as 'not bad enough' for action by the Regulator, yet not 'good enough' for patients and professional colleagues in a local service to have confidence in them. There is thus a significant 'regulatory gap' and it is this gap that endangers patient safety. (DoH, 2006)

There were a number of public consultations on the concept of 'revalidation' as a means of closing this 'regulatory gap'. The first step towards this process was the requirement since November 2009 that to practise, a doctor must not only be registered, but must also have a licence to practise. Without that licence, it is a criminal offence to practise medicine, write prescriptions, sign death certificates or undertake any other activities which are restricted to doctors holding a licence.

In late 2012, the GMC opened the process of 'revalidation' whereby every five years a doctor's licence to practise must be renewed. To do that, the doctor must be able to positively demonstrate to his 'Responsible Officer' that he is up to date and remains fit to practise.

It is envisaged that every organization providing healthcare will nominate a senior practising doctor to be the GMC's Responsible Officer. He is likely to be the organization's Medical Director. He has statutory duties to the GMC and so will be the bridge crossing the gap between local clinical governance and the GMC. His duties will be to ensure that there are adequate local systems for responding to concerns about a doctor, to oversee annual appraisals for all medical staff and to make recommendations for revalidation. He will write a report on the suitability of doctors in his organization for revalidation, based on their annual appraisals over the previous five years, and on any other information drawn from clinical governance systems. Where, as a result of his submissions, the GMC's Registrar considers withdrawing a doctor's licence, he will inform the doctor and give him 28 days to make representations about it. The Registrar must take those representations into account before making a decision. If he does then decide to withdraw the licence, the doctor will have the right to appeal to a Registration Appeals Panel. Equally, the GMC may well decide to put the matter through its Fitness to Practise Procedures.

What does this mean in practice for the individual doctor? He must keep a portfolio of supporting information for his annual appraisal, showing how he is keeping up to date, evaluating the quality of his work and recording feedback from colleagues and patients. The Royal Colleges for the different medical specialities will advise on the kind of material to be compiled.

The appraiser may also decide to use confidential questionnaires of patients and colleagues.

The GMC has warned practitioners that appraisal discussions will be more than a mere question of collating material. 'Your appraiser will want to know what you did with the supporting information, not just that you collected it.' The doctor will be expected to reflect on how he intends to develop and modify his practice.

Discussions at appraisals may be guided by the principles of the GMC's Good Medical Practice, which have been helpfully reduced into what are called The 'Four Domains', each domain having three 'Attributes'.

The theory is that a doctor who falls short of any of the required Twelve Attributes should be picked up by the clinical governance system during the five-year licence cycle, and given the appropriate support, so that his licence will be renewed at the end of the cycle.

The GMC says this about the closure of the 'regulatory gap':

'For the first time, employers, through Responsible Officers, will be required to make a positive statement about the Fitness to Practise of the doctors they employ. With their new responsibilities for overseeing revalidation, employers are more important than ever in promoting high standards of medical practice.'

Critics of the scheme say that a revalidation scheme based on the collection of papers and an annual appraisal will not effectively detect rogue doctors. They say that Shipman would have had his licence renewed. Critics also say that the scheme places too much power and influence in the hands of one person, the Medical Director/Responsible Officer, a feature which will draw the GMC into the politics of the workplace.

## (b) Consensual disposal

Ever since the procedural reforms of 2004, the GMC, sensitive to the criticism that doctors only ever look after their own, has placed a lot of emphasis on the transparency of its procedures. Decisions about impairment and about sanction are made in public at the conclusion of a public hearing (unless the issues under consideration concern a doctor's health in which case the hearing is in private). This is intended to maintain public confidence in the profession.

However, what has tended to happen is that after several days of exhausting and stressful evidence, although facts may have been proven against the doctor, it turns out that he can show insight and remediation. His Fitness to Practise may have been impaired at the time, but it is now no longer impaired. In that case, there is no finding of impairment and the worst that can happen is a warning. Was the hearing worth it?

Add to that the rising number of complaints, the rising number of hearings every year and the rising cost, and we find that the GMC is now thinking about dealing with at least some of its cases in a different way. The phrase 'consensual disposal' has been coined for the suggestion that the GMC and the doctor engage in some discussion about agreeing a sanction without the need for a hearing or witnesses. But would this kind of process undermine public confidence and create a perception of deals done 'behind closed doors'?

A recent consultation showed a large measure of support for the idea in principle. It was thought it might be most suitable for cases where there was no significant dispute about the facts. But it was also considered that there would be some cases in which such a process would be inappropriate, although it was difficult to establish what kind of cases these might be. More detailed proposals on the idea are now being developed by the GMC.

## 8   The role of the doctor

It is a term of all NHS employment contracts that staff must assist with investigations. Likewise, it is a professional requirement of the GMC's Good Medical Practice. A doctor who is asked to provide a written statement of events as part of any investigation– whether an internal hospital inquiry or a coroner's inquiry-must cooperate. Equally, he must be very conscious that what he writes now may be referred to in later proceedings. He therefore needs to be accurate. If there is any risk of trouble in the future, a doctor would be well advised to contact his MDO and ask for his proposed statement to be looked over by a medico-legal adviser.

### Witness statements

A doctor who is asked to prepare a witness statement concerning the care of a patient should always be provided with a copy of the relevant set of patient records to assist him.

Although a witness statement should be prepared as soon as possible after the event, so that the details are fresh in the mind, the doctor should not allow himself to be rushed. Accuracy is more important.

Here are some tips on writing a well laid out and clear witness statement:

### Formal requirements

- Write on one side of the paper only
- Type the statement and bind it using one staple in the top left-hand corner. Have a decent left and right margin and double space the document.
- Use a heading to orientate the reader e.g. Statement of Bob Smith following the death of Augustus Clark on E Ward at Pilkington Hospital on 22 November 2006.
- Number the pages and identify the statement in the top right-hand corner of each page, e.g. Page 2 Witness Statement of Bob SMITH.
- Number paragraphs and appendices.
- Refer to documents and names in capitals and express numbers as figures.
- Attach copies of protocols or other documents referred to, e.g. staff rota or clinical observations chart.
- Use narrative form and chronological order. Sign and date it.
- End with a statement of truth: 'I believe that the contents of this statement are true.'
- Spell-check the statement.

### Content

- Before starting, decide 'What are the issues?'
- Write a chronology. This will provide the structure.

- In the first paragraph, witnesses should set out who they are, their occupation and where they work (currently and at the time of the incident). It is important to orientate the reader, so a short CV is helpful. In more complex cases a fuller CV can be appended.
- There should be a main heading and subheadings.
- Use short sentences (a sentence that goes on for more than 2 lines is too long) and paragraphs (no more than 3 sentences per paragraph).
- Do not stray into another witness's evidence.
- Statements should contain no retrospective opinions, only contemporaneous opinions. Avoid statements like 'I thought for years this was going to happen'. Contemporaneous opinions should be backed up by facts. When stating a professional opinion, e.g. a diagnosis, explain the thinking behind the opinion.
- Do not use jargon. If technical terms have to be used, consider the use of a glossary and/or diagrams. Try to make the statement accessible to a non-clinician.
- Avoid pseudo-legal language.
- Identify individuals as they are introduced to the narrative.
- Ambiguous expressions such as 'I would have done such and such' should be avoided. If the doctor does not recall what he did, he should say so clearly. If, based on his normal practice, he believes he did such and such, then this should be made clear too.

## Apologies

A formal complaint against a doctor may be resolved, or it may lead to one or more other, more demanding investigations.

Patients often say that if they had received a sincere personal apology from the doctor for their error, they would not have pursued a claim or other form of complaint. Indeed, the received wisdom is that a personal apology often does satisfy a patient and/or the family and may resolve the problem. However, this is not always the case. Often a doctor may quite justifiably believe that he should not be blamed for a poor outcome. Lawyers too, prefer to investigate claims in detail before admitting any shortcomings in the standard of care provided. If an apology phrased in such a way that admits fault has already been made, then this could prejudice the case and make it difficult to defend what may in fact be an eminently defensible case. The NHSLA have issued guidance to hospital Trusts on written apologies (NHS Litigation Authority, 2009).

Sometimes, the answer to the question whether a doctor should apologize or not will be obvious. For example, where there has been an obvious mistake in a medication dosage, a prompt apology may well be advisable. Sometimes it is not so obvious. The best advice to a doctor is to discuss the matter with his colleagues, his MDO and/or the Trust's complaints or legal manager.

# 9   **Presenting oral evidence**

Having looked at negligence claims, disciplinary hearings, coroner's hearings and GMC hearings, it is appropriate to say a few words about how to give evidence. For the way a witness presents his evidence affects the weight given to it by the court, inquiry or tribunal.

Remember that the role of the factual witness is to assist the Tribunal. He is not there to argue with the barrister.

Barristers may try to draw witnesses into an argument. They may also use other techniques to disconcert them, such as moving between multiple documents, repeating the same question is a slightly different way to try and elicit a different answer and pausing in the hope that the doctor will 'talk into the silence'. Once the witness recognizes that they are just techniques, they can watch out for them and so remain in control.

The lawyer is only doing his job. Witnesses have to separate themselves from the evidence and not get angry.

Before giving evidence, witnesses should:
- re-read and think about all the evidence including the records, protocols, national guidelines and professional standards;
- re-read witness statements and Court/Inquiry documents (if appropriate) and ask their lawyer to explain anything they do not understand;
- check with the lawyers whether there are any other documents they would like the witness to read, such as clinical studies;
- tell the lawyers about any mistakes or omissions in the witness statement;
- visit the courtroom beforehand; ask the Court for a tour;
- if possible see the Court/Inquiry 'in action' beforehand;
- plan the route to the hearing, arrange where to meet everyone and work out what to wear;
- exchange telephone numbers with the legal team;
- put the Court telephone number into their mobile phone;
- practise taking the oath and giving their credentials.

At the hearing:
- report to the reception desk where you will need to register;
- be prepared to come into contact with family members and media representatives;
- keep conversations to a minimum and nonverbal communications appropriate;
- on entering the courtroom sit down and do not talk;
- stand up when the judge or panel arrives and then be seated;
- the proceedings will be recorded; be prepared to speak clearly and slowly;
- pause before answering any questions;
- listen carefully to the question;

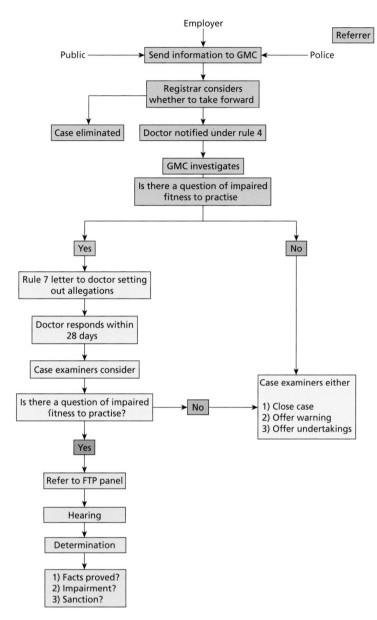

**Figure 3.1** Fitness to practise procedure – a summary.

- deliver your answers to the judge or panel; the best way to ensure this is to stand with your feet facing the judge or panel and turn from the hips to take questions from the lawyers;
- try to keep answers to questions brief and to the point;
- try to eliminate passion from your answers.

No-one, not even a seasoned expert witness, enjoys the stress of giving evidence. But to do so is part of a doctor's professional duty.

## 10 Emotional repercussions

Many doctors take criticism extremely personally, even if the complaint or claim is relatively straightforward and can be put to rest without too much difficulty. Each doctor will react differently. The experience may leave them feeling injured and cynical. Some may find that the complaint or claim takes a physical toll on them. Some may even leave the profession altogether. Others seem able to take a relaxed attitude towards a claim, at least on the surface.

Stress associated with complaints and claims can lead to anxiety, depression and on rare occasions even suicide. People deal with stress in different ways, but talking to friends and family can help. The solicitor and the medico-legal advisor at a doctor's MDO are on hand to help and to listen to concerns. They are there to provide emotional support as much as legal advice.

The British Medical Association also offers a 24-hour counselling service with the opportunity to talk to a counsellor or a doctor on 08459 200 169. A doctor may need the help of a GP, psychotherapist or psychiatrist. Some Deaneries, such as the London Deanery, offer free emotional support and psychotherapy to doctors suffering from stress or emotional ill health. Doctors can refer themselves to this service. In London the service (called MedNet) is run by Consultant Psychiatrists (0208 938 2411).

## 11 Conclusion

We hope that this final part of the book has clarified the procedures which may come into play after a medical error. The reader may well be daunted by the number of parallel investigations which can be made in relation to a single error. However he should take heart. High quality professional help is available from his hospital Trust and MDO. Our advice is to make full use of it.

The other point to make is that error is part of the human condition. In 2011 there were 8781 complaints to the GMC and it is thus not uncommon for a doctor to be referred. All doctors make mistakes, even excellent ones and even those who sit on GMC Fitness to Practise Panels. Doctors who make mistakes may become better at their jobs as a result. They can, and do, go on to have successful and productive careers. The key is to reflect on errors and pay heed to any lessons that can be learnt.

## References

Department of Health (2006) Good doctors, safer patients: Proposals to strengthen the system to assure and improve the performance of doctors and to protect the safety of patients.

The Local Authorities Social Services and NHS Complaints (England) Regulations 2009.

NHS Litigation Authority (2009) *Apologies and Explanations.*
www.nhsla.com/NR/rdonlyres/00F14BA6-0621-4A23-B885-
   FA18326FF745/0/ApologiesandExplanations.pdf.   Last   accessed   30
   May 2012.
Scally G, Donaldson L (1998) Clinical governance and the drive for quality
   improvement in the new NHS in England. *BMJ* **317**: 61–5.

# Index

*Avoiding Errors in Adult Medicine*, First Edition. Ian P. Reckless, D. John M. Reynolds,
Sally Newman, Joseph E. Raine, Kate Williams and Jonathan Bonser.
© 2013 John Wiley & Sons, Ltd. Published 2013 by John Wiley & Sons, Ltd.